BRETT BLUMENTHAL

GET REAL AND STOP DIETING!

FORGET THE FADS, LEARN THE FACTS, AND FEEL FABULOUS

PUBLISHED BY

Published by AmazonEncore
P.O. Box 400818
Las Vegas, NV 89140

ISBN-13: 9781935597292
ISBN-10: 1935597299

To my best friend and mom:
you have given me wings to fly,
and the love and support to keep them flapping.

I love you more than words.

WHAT THEY'RE SAYING ABOUT *GET REAL...*

"Where other books offer quick-fix dieting fads, Brett Blumenthal offers a refreshing approach to healthy eating as a lifestyle. Whether you've been dieting for years or are already on a path to healthy living, *GET REAL* is a fantastic resource that's relevant for a lifetime."

—Lauren Mackler - Author of the international bestseller
Solemate: Master the Art of Aloneness & Transform Your Life

"GET REAL is a refreshingly pragmatic and easy guide to leading a healthier lifestyle. It's the 'diet book' for people who hate diet books!"

—Andrew Brooks - Founder, Gnu Foods

"Obesity is the number one health problem in the United States today. It leads to heart disease, hypertension, diabetes, and atherosclerosis, and has been implicated in the development of cancer. Simply put, it is a major killer! While many people want to lose weight and try a wide variety of 'fad diets,' most dieters fail at dieting or regain the lost weight once they achieve their goal. *GET REAL and STOP Dieting!* offers a no-nonsense approach to a healthy lifestyle that will make a huge difference to anyone who follows its precepts. Ms. Blumenthal has done a superb job of demystifying the subject and presenting, in lay terminology, facts and strategies that make healthy eating understandable, possible, and…yes…even enjoyable."

—*William H. Koch, M.D.*

"Brett Blumenthal's approach to a healthier and leaner body is presented in a straightforward, no-nonsense way. *GET REAL and STOP Dieting!* shows you how to 'keep it natural' while keeping it simple!"

—*Pete Cerqua - Author of* The 90-Second Fitness Solution

"Insightful, clear, and concise! Brett Blumenthal's *GET REAL and STOP Dieting!* is a wonderful guide to better health."

—*Alex Ong - Professional Speaker and Author of* Mind Your Own Wellness

ACKNOWLEDGEMENTS

I would like to express my sincere thanks to all of the individuals who have contributed to helping make *GET REAL and STOP Dieting!* a true reality.

Thank you to Terry Goodman for being my advocate and for supporting me every step of the way. Having you in my corner has made this adventure quite enjoyable and fun.

A big thank you to Sarah Tomashek, who has been extremely patient and responsive in dealing with my type A tendencies throughout the marketing process. You're an angel!

To Jessica Smith and Ann Thrash, your meticulous attention to detail is nothing short of awe-inspiring. Thank you for being so diligent and thorough. You are miracle workers!

Abby Harris, thank you for your tenacity in dealing with road blocks as they surfaced. You paved the way for a smoother ride.

Thank you to the team at AmazonEncore for your time, dedication, and effort in making this possible. You've done an amazing job!

To my research assistant, Sarah Schumacher: thank you for your resourcefulness, your enthusiasm, and your genuine passion for the topic and the project. Your efforts made *GET REAL* the fact-based resource that we wanted it to be.

To Lynne Morgan: thank you for your creativity and unique concoctions. They gave the recipe section more flair and pizzazz…not to mention mouthwatering flavor!

A thank you to Stacy Kennedy for your support and expertise in helping ensure that the content was current, appropriate, and relevant to the topic at hand.

David, thank you for your constant encouragement, love, and support in my endeavors, and for chasing dreams with me. And thank you to Mom and Bill for your unconditional love and belief in me. I love you all and feel blessed to have you in my life and in my corner.

CONTENTS

FOREWORD

Adopting healthy eating habits is one of the most important personal choices we can make to better our health and well-being. The philosophy of striving for a plant-based diet consisting of minimally processed foods is well supported by a wealth of research from around the world. Many Americans understand that eating healthy foods is important and have a good sense of what those foods are. Yet, somehow, making healthy eating work in our everyday lives has become an unattainable mystery. Good common sense seems to have been replaced with media hype over the latest diet craze or "magic" food. However, a healthy diet is truly a healthy diet. Whether you want to lose weight, look great, increase your energy, or manage or prevent chronic diseases such as diabetes, heart disease, and cancer, the same basic principles of healthy eating apply.

Generations ago, eating was much less complicated. We tended to shop more often at markets that provided fresh, locally produced foods. Families ate together, and most meals were cooked and eaten at home. Today, with the prevalence of packaged convenience foods and easy access to cheaper food in restaurants, our waistlines are expanding and our wellness is declining rapidly.

A study published in 2005[1] in the journal *Archives of Internal Medicine* revealed that the percentage of Americans who:

- don't smoke was 76 percent;
- maintain a healthy weight was 40 percent;
- eat five or more servings of fruits and vegetables a day was 23 percent;

- engage in physical activity for at least thirty minutes five days a week was 22 percent.

The most staggering conclusion of this study was that the percentage of people who were assimilating *all four behaviors* was a mere 3 percent.

A European study, published in the same journal in September 2009,[2] compared participants who adhered to all four of the above behaviors to those who did not. It found that the first group (who never smoked; maintained a BMI [body mass index] below 30; ate a healthy diet of fruits, vegetables, and whole grains with limited meat consumption; and got 3.5 hours or more of physical activity per week) had a:

- 93 percent lower chance of developing diabetes;
- 81 percent lower risk of heart attack;
- 50 percent lower risk of stroke;
- 36 percent lower risk of developing cancer.

There is clearly a need for practical, easy, reasonable ways to change our behaviors to those that promote health.

For many, losing weight means dieting and dieting equals misery: full of restriction, bad-tasting food, giving up the foods we love, and alienation from friends and family who eat "regular food." Brett's book *GET REAL and STOP Dieting!* is a fresh approach to losing weight and improving wellness. This easy-to-read guide is full of good, scientific information about nutrition and wellness, and plenty of practical tools to apply the information into execution. With such a huge discrepancy between the known benefits of a healthy lifestyle and the number of Americans able to implement the behaviors needed, *GET REAL and STOP Dieting!* helps to fill this gap. The book's recipes and tips for label reading are valuable assets for beginners as well as for those who have already been working to eat healthy for years.

Brett breaks down complicated information into easy-to-read charts and shopping lists to guide your next grocery store trip. And although Brett is not a nutritionist, her book promotes a philosophy that nutrition professionals and the general public can support. The information is well researched and uses up-to-date scientific parameters to back the recommendations and tips included in this book. I look forward to recommending *GET REAL and STOP Dieting!* to my clients.

Stacy Kennedy, MPH, RD, CSO, LDN
Senior Clinical Nutritionist
Brigham & Women's Hospital
Boston, Massachusetts

References:

1. M. J. Reeves and A. P. Rafferty, "Healthy Lifestyle Characteristics Among Adults in the United States, 2000," *Arch Intern Med.* 2005;165:854–857.

2. E. S. Ford, M. M. Bergmann, J. Kroger, A. Schienkiewitz, C. Weikert, and H. Boeing, "Healthy Living Is the Best Revenge: Findings from the European Prospective Investigation into Cancer and Nutrition–Potsdam Study," *Arch Intern Med.* 2009;169(15):1355–1362.

INTRODUCTION

Let's face it: there's a ton of information out there about dieting, nutrition, and weight loss, and often a lot of it isn't very helpful. You have to weed through tons of articles, blogs, Web sites and health magazines to get to the nuggets of information that are most important, most accurate, and most helpful. Further, much of that information is contradictory.

Every which way you turn, there's a new study on something you should or shouldn't be eating, what will or won't cause cancer, what will or won't help you lose weight, what will or won't burn fat. It is enough to drive anyone crazy! No wonder eating healthy seems complicated and, maybe, even impossible. I know that the more complex something seems, the less I'm interested in it...let alone inspired to follow it.

Thanks to bombardment from the media, unscrupulous false advertising, and countless fad diets, it's hard to imagine that healthy eating can be easy. But it can be. In this book, you'll discover an approach to eating that I like to call "GET REAL." It utilizes five basic principles that are founded in facts, not fads. As a result, you'll have the framework to help you eat healthy today, tomorrow, and for the rest of your life. And there's an added bonus: you will automatically shed excess pounds and, with surprising ease, maintain a healthy weight for a lifetime.

THE FIVE "GET REAL" PRINCIPLES

1. KEEP IT WHOLE, KEEP IT NATURAL, KEEP IT SIMPLE
2. FOCUS ON FIBER
3. PACK LEAN PROTEINS INTO EVERY MEAL
4. ENJOY HEALTHY FATS
5. EAT SMALL, OFTEN, AND MINDFULLY

In the following chapters, we'll discuss these five principles in detail, including the meaning and importance of each and, perhaps most critical, how to implement them both easily and effectively. So forget the fads and get ready to look and feel fabulous!

Setting Things Straight

Whether you're fifteen or fifty, there's a chance you've acquired some preconceived ideas about healthy eating and what it actually entails. So before we address our five principles, let's take a moment to explore and debunk five commonly held misconceptions.

Misconception 1: If you eat healthy, you must be on a diet.

This one never fails to amuse and amaze! Too often, the word "diet" is confused with the concept of dieting. Most people equate the word with deprivation, especially as related to foods they love. Whether you are at your ideal weight or trying to lose weight, eating healthy is NOT dieting. It IS eating a healthy diet, which is a proactive lifestyle choice. If you want to eat healthy, you are choosing to do so. You choose to optimize the way you eat to look and feel your best.

Misconception 2: Eating healthy is boring, tastes awful, and is never satisfying.

Truth be told, eating healthy can taste better, can be wonderfully varied, and can fill you up for longer periods of time than food that is unhealthy. Many individuals who make a long-term switch to a healthier diet swear that they don't miss the unhealthy foods they once ate. Some actually find them distasteful! As you eat quality foods, your cravings for those that are bad for you and lack nutritional value will diminish.

Misconception 3: There is a secret to weight loss.

There is absolutely no secret, no magic pill, and no trick to losing weight. You are an individual with individual needs. As a result, fad diets and "secret weight-loss programs" may work for some, but not necessarily for others. That said, regardless of what diets you have followed in the past, there's a good chance they incorporated at least three out of the five principles presented in this book. Why? Because certain rules always apply to healthy eating.

Misconception 4: You need to count calories to be successful.

Although food journaling is advisable, it isn't necessary. For the most part, calorie counting is a must for those people who don't follow the five "eating healthy" principles. It's when we stray that we need to count and track what we ingest, because we're consuming a lot of empty calories that provide very little, if any, nutrition. The five principles, however, will deliver an easy-to-follow guide so that you feel full and satisfied without the need for counting calories. Just think: you'll be able to spend time doing the things you enjoy most!

Misconception 5: Eating healthy is difficult and complicated.

Eating a healthy diet is not rocket science. It never has been and it never will be. Don't tell the experts this, but you don't need a degree in nutrition, a PhD, or an MD to eat well. All you need is a basic, easy-to-implement framework that will demystify the realm of healthy eating and provide simple, commonsense rules that are easy to remember and easy to put into action.

The "GET REAL" principles will address each and every one of these misconceptions head-on. So if you're ready to learn about the "GET REAL" approach to eating healthy for life, get out your knife and fork and STOP dieting!

PART 1

THE "GET REAL" PRINCIPLES

1

KEEP IT WHOLE, KEEP IT NATURAL, KEEP IT SIMPLE

This is the foundation on which all "GET REAL" principles are built. Leading nutrition authorities claim that consuming whole foods is the most effective dietary approach. The more whole, natural foods you eat, the better off you will be. This means consuming foods that are not processed and do not contain preservatives, chemicals, fillers, or artificial flavors or colors.

WHAT IS A WHOLE FOOD?

A whole food, by its truest definition, is found in nature and can be eaten or cooked as you find it. Foods that grow in the soil, on a tree, or come directly from animals, fish or fowl, are whole foods. If, however, they have to be refined in a manufacturing plant to reach their edible state or they include additives (chemicals, preservatives, coloring, or flavoring), they are not whole foods.

Not every packaged food is refined or manufactured. Brown rice is a typical example. It is extracted from the plant and packaged for the convenience of storing and selling. Similarly, a packaged food that contains multiple ingredients may be considered "whole" if each ingredient is whole by itself. Trail mix, for example, can be whole if it combines three whole foods (nuts, raisins, and seeds). On the other hand, there are products, such as instant oatmeal, that may seem to be whole but actually contain extra sugars and additives.

The best way to know if a packaged food is truly whole is to read the list of ingredients. If you can pronounce all of them AND you know what they are, the packaged food is most likely close to whole. Further, whole foods DO NOT contain added sugars, salt, or fat.

WHY ARE WHOLE FOODS IMPORTANT?

1. **Whole foods are lower in calories.** When comparing a whole version of a food with a processed version, more often than not, the whole version will be lower in calories. Whole foods have no add-ons that represent empty, unwanted calories. They come as nature made them, without added fat, sugar, or sodium. By increasing your whole food intake, you will cut down on unnecessary ingredients and calories inherent to processed and fast foods.

2. **Whole foods are more filling.** Whole foods are nutrient dense, which makes them very filling and satisfying. When foods undergo processing, they lose fiber together with other nutrients that appease your appetite. White rice, for example, is made by stripping fiber from brown rice. Without the fiber, the white rice loses its ability to fill you up. So you eat more or feel hungry sooner than you would had you eaten the brown rice.

3. **Whole foods protect against disease.** Whole foods contain vitamins and minerals, antioxidants, phenolics, fiber, and other phytochemicals. According to the American Institute for Cancer Research (AICR), these nutrients help lower the

risk of certain diseases, including cancer, heart disease, high blood pressure, and diabetes. On the other hand, ingredients included in processed foods may contribute to these diseases.

4. **Whole foods are pure.** Whole foods don't contain chemicals, preservatives, or additives that can be harmful to your health, whereas many add-ons found in processed foods raise a serious eyebrow. Some are considered carcinogens (substances known to cause cancer); others have caused allergic reactions; still others can interfere with the body's functions and metabolism.

5. **Whole foods help decrease unhealthy fat consumption.** Incorporating whole foods in your diet makes it infinitely easier to avoid "bad-for-you" fats (trans fats and saturated fats). These are often added to processed foods or are created during the cooking process of manufactured and fast foods.

Did You Know?

A research study reported that when switching from a refined-food diet to an unrefined-food diet, women ate 61% less saturated fat.

READING INGREDIENT LISTS FOR WHOLE FOODS

The ability to read nutrition labels is the key to understanding whether or not a food is whole. The following two examples compare and contrast ingredient lists for whole versus processed forms of common foods. Ingredients in bold type are obvious giveaways that the product has additives, is processed, or is refined.

Maple and Brown Sugar Instant oatmeal *processed*	**Old-Fashioned Rolled Oats** *whole*
Ingredients: Whole Grain Rolled Oats (with oat bran), **Sugar, Natural and Artificial Flavors, Salt, Calcium Carbonate, Guar Gum,** Oat Flour, **Caramel Color, Niacinamide, Vitamin A Palmitate, Reduced Iron, Pyridoxine Hydrochloride, Riboflavin, Thiamin Mononitrate, Folic Acid.**	**Ingredients:** 100% Natural Whole Grain Rolled Oats.

In the maple and brown sugar instant oatmeal example, sugar, artificial flavors, salt, calcium carbonate, guar gum, and coloring, among others, are added ingredients. The old-fashioned rolled oats, however, contain 100 percent natural whole grain rolled oats. Chances are you know what rolled oats are, but you very well may not know or have heard of guar gum or calcium carbonate. This is a good indication that the oatmeal is processed. And although some of these added ingredients are vitamins (pyridoxine hydrochloride), they are added as a result of processing.

Chicken Breast Nuggets	**Fresh Chicken Breast**
processed	*whole*

Ingredients: Boneless Chicken Breast With Rib Meat, Water, **Potassium Lactate, Sodium Lactate, Salt, Sodium Phosphates, Sodium Diacetate, Flavoring.** Breaded With: **Bleached Wheat Flour,** Water, **Enriched Bleached Wheat Flour (Enriched With Niacin, Reduce Iron, Thiamine Mononitrate, Riboflavin, Folic Acid),** Yellow Corn Flour, Yellow Corn Meal, **Dextrose,** Dried Whey, **Salt, Sugar, Potassium Sorbate (to Protect Freshness),** Spice, **Soybean Oil, Calcium Propionate (to Protect Freshness), Guar Gum, Flavoring,** Extractives of Paprika (Color), Spice Extractive.

Ingredients: Chicken Breast; Natural Chicken Broth (Chicken Broth, **Salt, Carrageenan**).*

* When you buy meat, it's often sold in its own juices or a derivative of its own juices to keep it moist and extend shelf life.

In looking at the chicken breast nuggets label, you see tons of additives, including bleached wheat flour, soybean oil, dextrose, and sugar, all of which are far from natural to chicken. And although the fresh chicken breast has salt and carrageenan to preserve freshness, these two ingredients are nothing in comparison to those of the nuggets.

WHAT ARE THE BEST SOURCES OF WHOLE FOODS?

Fresh and frozen vegetables and fruits, unrefined grains, legumes and beans, nuts, seeds, eggs, and ocean-raised fish are all excellent whole food sources. Butcher-cut poultry and meat, although "handled and packaged," can also be considered whole. Be aware, however, that most poultry and meats are packaged in their own juices to extend shelf life and to preserve moisture.

WHAT FOODS SHOULD I AVOID?

Rule of thumb: Avoid processed or manufactured foods. The worst offenders include:

- **Refined Sugar and Sweetened Foods.** Avoid foods with refined sugars as well as high-fructose and regular corn syrups. Candy, soda, syrup, jelly, cookies, and baked goods are on the "avoid list." Instead, eat foods that are naturally sweet or sweetened with fruit or 100 percent fruit juice. You can also use natural sweeteners, such as honey or agave nectar.

- **White Flour, Refined Flour, Enriched Flour.** Avoid eating bread, cereal, or grain products that have been processed, refined, or bleached, e.g., those that use white flour, refined flour, or enriched flour. During the milling process, refined flour loses key vitamins and nutrients in the germ and bran. As a result, manufacturers will enrich flours by adding certain B vitamins and iron back into the flour after processing. Fiber (an important nutrient), however, is not added back to enriched flour.

WHOLE GRAINS VS. WHOLE FOODS

Don't confuse whole grains with whole foods. Any food made from wheat, rice, oats, cornmeal, barley, or another cereal grain is a GRAIN product. For example, old-fashioned rolled oats, as we discussed earlier, contain 100% WHOLE GRAINS…or whole oats. Instant oatmeal also contains whole grains…or old-fashioned rolled oats…however, it contains other ingredients and additives that take it out of the WHOLE FOOD category.

- **Packaged Foods with "Un-Whole" Ingredients.** Many packaged foods that seem healthy contain fillers, preservatives, and other ingredients you don't want in your diet. If you do choose something that has been manufactured (anything canned, packaged, etc.), try to avoid those that contain ingredients you don't recognize or those we list on the "Added Ingredients to Avoid" chart provided later in this chapter.

- **Diet Foods.** Diet foods are lower-calorie versions of their high-calorie cousins, made by reducing the sugar and/or fat content. Reduced-sugar foods and beverages are often loaded with highly processed, chemically derived sugar substitutes; reduced-fat foods usually have a lot of added sugars. Both options require the very additives and processing that are best avoided. To understand "diet food" labels, refer to the "Diet Food Labels" chart on the next page.

Did You Know?

Studies show low-fat labels can lead people to overeat snack foods by changing perception of serving size and decreasing guilt.

DIET FOOD LABELS

It's important to understand nutrient content claims on packaged diet foods. Claims can often be misleading.

Term	Example	What It Really Means
Free	• Sugar-Free • Fat-Free	• No amount of or only a minimal amount of the nutrient makes up the food
Less	• Less Sugar • Less Fat	• Nutritionally altered to contain at least 25% less of the nutrient or calories than the referenced food
Light	• Light Cream Cheese	• Contains one-third fewer calories or half the fat of the referenced food; if the food derives 50% or more calories from fat, the reduction must be 50% or more
Low	• Low-Fat • Low-Sodium	• May be used on foods that can be eaten frequently without exceeding dietary guidelines; amount varies depending on nutrient
Reduced	• Reduced-Fat • Reduced-Sugar	• Interchangeable with "less" • Nutritionally altered to contain at least 25% less of the nutrient or calories than the referenced food • If sugar is reduced, it does not mean that it is sugar-free

ARTIFICIAL SWEETENERS AND WEIGHT

A long-term study of nearly 3,700 residents of San Antonio, Texas, showed that those who averaged three or more artificially sweetened beverages per day were more likely to gain weight over an eight-year period than those who didn't drink artificially sweetened beverages. Further, research conducted at Purdue University found rats that ate food sweetened with saccharin, an artificial sweetener, took in more calories and gained more weight than rats fed sugar-sweetened food.

Beyond weight gain, artificial sweeteners continue to conjure much controversy in regards to health and disease. To be safe, it is best to avoid artificial sweeteners and, if possible, cut them out of your diet altogether.

- **Fried Foods.** Fried foods, especially those that are packaged or come from fast food restaurants, more often than not contain saturated and trans fats. These fats have been linked to disease and other health problems.

- **Fast Foods.** As upsetting as this may be, fast foods are, by all measures, the worst of the worst offenders. Most are mass produced, processed, and filled with preservatives, artificial flavorings, colorings, and other additives. Furthermore, fast food restaurants tend to use ingredients of lesser quality combined with unhealthy fats.

ADDED INGREDIENTS TO AVOID

Ingredient	Why It Is Used	Why It Is Bad
Artificial Colors	• Chemical compounds made from coal-tar derivatives to enhance color	• Linked to allergic reactions, fatigue, asthma, skin rashes, hyperactivity, and headaches
Artificial Flavorings	• Cheap chemical mixtures that mimic natural flavors	• Linked to allergic reactions, dermatitis, eczema, hyperactivity, and asthma • Can affect enzymes, RNA, and thyroid
Artificial Sweeteners **(Acesulfame-K, Aspartame, Equal, NutraSweet, Saccharin, Sweet'n Low, Sucralose, Splenda, Sorbitol)**	• Highly processed, chemically derived, zero-calorie sweeteners found in diet foods and diet products to reduce calories per serving	• Can negatively impact metabolism • Some have been linked to cancer, dizziness, hallucinations, and headaches
Benzoate Preservatives (BHT, BHA, TBHQ)	• Compounds that preserve fats and prevent them from becoming rancid	• May result in hyperactivity, angioedema, asthma, rhinitis, dermatitis, tumors, and urticaria • Can affect estrogen balance and levels
Brominated Vegetable Oil **(BVO)**	• Chemical that boosts flavor in many citric-based fruit and soft drinks	• Increases triglycerides and cholesterol • Can damage liver, testicles, thyroid, heart, and kidneys

Ingredient	Why It Is Used	Why It Is Bad
High-Fructose Corn Syrup **(HFCS)**	• Cheap alternative to cane and beet sugar • Sustains freshness in baked goods • Blends easily in beverages to maintain sweetness	• May predispose the body to turn fructose into fat • Increases risk for Type 2 diabetes, coronary heart disease, stroke, and cancer • Isn't easily metabolized by the liver
MSG **(Monosodium Glutamate)**	• Flavor enhancer in restaurant food, salad dressing, chips, frozen entrees, soups, and other foods	• May stimulate appetite and cause headaches, nausea, weakness, wheezing, edema, change in heart rate, burning sensations, and difficulty in breathing
Olestra	• An indigestible fat substitute used primarily in foods that are fried and baked	• Inhibits absorption of some nutrients • Linked to gastrointestinal disease, diarrhea, gas, cramps, bleeding, and incontinence
Shortening, Hydrogenated, and Partially Hydrogenated Oils **(Palm, Soybean, and Others)**	• Industrially created fats used in more than 40,000 food products in the United States • Cheaper than most other oils	• Contain high levels of trans fats, which raise bad cholesterol and lower good cholesterol, contributing to risk of heart disease
Sodium Nitrite and Nitrate	• Preserves, colors, and flavors cured meats and fish • Prevents botulism	• Can combine with chemicals in stomach to form nitrosamine—a known carcinogen

HOW SHOULD I INCORPORATE WHOLE FOODS INTO MY DIET?

Obviously, there are times when we can't eat whole, all-natural foods. But whenever possible, it is best to eat those that are closest to their natural state. Again, if the food is packaged, make sure you check the label for ingredients to avoid. Here are some tips:

- **Fruit.** Eat fruit raw or in homemade smoothies. Avoid fruit sauces (e.g., applesauce), fruit cocktails, and fruit snacks; they often have added sugars and other ingredients. Further, a whole fruit is a better choice than a fruit drink or juice. Fruit juices have less fiber and more calories than whole fruits. For example, one 6-ounce serving of orange juice has 85 calories and 0 grams of fiber, while a medium orange has just 65 calories and 3 grams of fiber.

- **Vegetables.** Although you may have heard that raw vegetables are better than cooked, each vegetable has its own individual preferred cooking method. Further, some nutrients are enhanced by cooking, while others are lost. As a result, it is best to eat a variety of vegetables, prepared in a variety of ways, to be sure you get all of the nutrients they provide.

- **Meat, Poultry, and Fish.** Fresh cuts of meat, poultry, and fish from the meat or fish counters—instead of the frozen food aisle—are best. Try to eliminate processed, packaged meats that contain a list of ingredients other than the meat itself: e.g., hot dogs, lunch meat, sausages, chopped meat, chicken nuggets, or chicken fingers. Aim for the leanest cuts/parts to avoid high amounts of saturated fat. Grill, bake, or broil to eliminate fatty oils used in frying or heavy sautéing.

COOKING VEGETABLES: NUTRITIONAL VALUES

A study from the Universities of Parma and Naples found that boiling carrots, zucchini, and broccoli decreased their vitamin C concentrations, implying that the vitamin is damaged or harmed by heat or boiling. However, the opposite occurred in regards to other antioxidants. When boiling carrots, for example, the concentration of vitamin C decreased by 9%. However, the concentration of carotenoid (another antioxidant) significantly increased. And although boiling or steaming vegetables decreases their vitamin C content, microwaving results in only a slight reduction in vitamin C levels.

- **Whole Grains and Legumes.** Aim for 100 percent whole grains whenever possible. This includes 100 percent whole wheat, brown rice, quinoa, bulgur, oats, rye, and barley. If you choose to eat pastas, look for those that list whole wheat or other whole grains first on the ingredient list. Canned or dried beans are good as well.

- **Keep It Fresh.** Eat foods that are fresh whenever possible. The fresher the foods, the more nutrients they deliver, while packaged foods, with additives and/or preservatives, are lower in nutrients than their fresh counterparts. Avoid produce and meats that are canned or jarred, especially those packaged in sauces, syrups, or other preservatives. If vegetables or fruit are out of season, frozen may be a better choice than produce shipped from far away. Be sure, however, to look for choices that are free of other ingredients and are loose in the bag (not clumped together).

SPOTTING "REAL" WHOLE GRAINS

At a minimum, it is recommended that you consume 48 grams of whole grain ingredients per day, with one serving established as 16 grams. Unfortunately, many products contain both whole grains AND refined grains. Consequently, the Whole Grains Council (WGC) initiated two stamps in 2005 to help consumers find products containing whole grains.

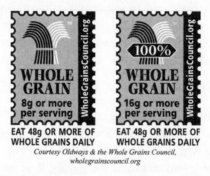

EAT 48g OR MORE OF   EAT 48g OR MORE OF
WHOLE GRAINS DAILY   WHOLE GRAINS DAILY

Courtesy Oldways & the Whole Grains Council,
wholegrainscouncil.org

The "Whole Grain Stamp" on the left is used to identify those products that contain at least 8 grams of whole grains per serving. The "100% Whole Grain Stamp," on the right is applied to products that are made with 100 percent whole grains and provide one serving or more (at least 16 grams) of whole grains per serving.

If a food doesn't have a WGC stamp, look to see if it contains **100 percent** whole wheat, brown rice, oats, oatmeal, or wheat berries... or lists a whole grain or stone-ground whole grain in the ingredient list. Steer clear of those foods that contain degerminated bran or wheat germ, or enriched flour. And those products that contain wheat flour, semolina, durum wheat, organic flour, or multigrains may or may not provide whole grains and, as a result, might be best if avoided. When in doubt, buy products with the WGC stamps: they are the best indicators of exactly how whole the products are, which takes the guesswork out of the selection process.

- **Farmers' Markets.** Farmers' markets are a great way to get fresh food, support your local economy, and promote sustainability. Farmers' markets tend to carry fresh, homegrown, in-season produce, which translates to "far more delicious and nutritious" than supermarket selections. When foods are not locally grown, they often aren't in season and can lose their freshness factor during transportation. And since the food is brought in from local farms, less gas is needed for transport, resulting in less impact to the environment.

Did You Know?

A locavore eats only foods grown or harvested within a 100-mile radius of his or her home.

- **Organic.** If your store carries organic products and you can afford them, INDULGE—especially with meats and produce. Organic means no pesticides, hormones, or antibiotics, all of which may be harmful to your health. Remember, however, organic does not necessarily mean local or fresh.

LOCAL VS. IMPORTED PRODUCE

In a survey of five hundred consumers in the Northeast United States, 88% of consumers believed that local produce was fresher than imported produce; 60% believed that it looked better; and 62% believed that it tasted better.

- **Cooking.** Avoid frying and heavy sautéing: they require heavy use of oil and butter, which counteract the healthful benefits of eating whole foods. When sautéing, use no more than one tablespoon of olive oil or canola oil to coat the bottom of the pan. Better yet, use a low-sodium broth or water in place of oil.

- **Condiments.** Raw mustards, horseradish, spices, and vinegars add incredible flavor to dishes. Avoid off-the-shelf barbecue sauces, ketchup, and other prepared sauces when possible. They tend to contain sugar, high-fructose corn syrup, MSG, sodium, and other ingredients that may contain "empty" calories and are unnecessary and unhealthy.

More often than not, you can find a whole food option for a processed food. To demonstrate, we've included several examples in the "Food Substitutions: Processed vs. Whole" chart on the next page.

FOOD SUBSTITUTIONS: PROCESSED VS. WHOLE

NO!	Yes!! Yes!! Yes!!

Fried Chicken Fingers → Grilled Chicken Breast

French Fries → Roasted Potatoes

Sugared Cereals → Whole Grain Cereal

Vitamin Water → Water with Lemon

White Flour Bread → 100% Whole-Grain Bread

THE ONE-MINUTE SUMMARY

1. A whole food is found in nature, and although it might require cooking, it can be enjoyed without refining or manufacturing processes.
2. Whole foods are beneficial because they:
   - are more nutritious, lower in calories, and more filling than processed foods;
   - help fight disease;
   - are safer than refined or manufactured products;
   - contain far less unhealthy fats than refined foods.
3. Fruit, vegetables, nuts, seeds, eggs, fish, and unprocessed meats are the best sources of whole food.
4. Avoid eating:
   - foods with refined sugars and corn syrups;
   - diet foods;
   - fried or heavily sautéed foods;
   - foods made with refined or bleached flour;
   - packaged foods that contain "un-whole" ingredients;
   - fast foods.
5. Whenever possible, eat foods that are closest to their natural form.

2

FOCUS ON FIBER

At every meal and with every snack, incorporate fiber in your diet! The FDA recommends a minimum daily fiber intake of 25 grams; however, 25 to 35 grams a day is optimal.

WHAT IS FIBER?

Dietary fiber is found in carbohydrates (vegetables, fruit, beans, and grains) and includes all parts of the plant that your body can't absorb. Fiber is found mostly in the outer layer of plants, and unlike other food substances, your body doesn't digest it. Instead, it passes through your digestive tract without being broken down or changed. Fiber comes in two forms: insoluble, which doesn't dissolve in water, and soluble, which dissolves in water to form a gel-like substance.

WHY IS FIBER IMPORTANT?

1. **Fiber helps stabilize energy and sugar levels.** Because fiber slows digestion, it also helps to slow absorption of sugars into the bloodstream. Soluble fiber, specifically, delays the absorption of sugars and starches by dragging partly digested food through the intestine. This keeps your blood sugar, insulin, and energy levels more stable throughout the day.

2. **Fiber fills you up.** Fiber is a bulking agent that stays in the stomach longer, providing a greater sense of satisfaction between meals. For instance, a slice of 100 percent whole grain bread is more filling than two slices of white bread. Additionally, because fiber needs to be chewed thoroughly, it slows down the eating process. This helps prevent overeating: the brain has time to recognize that the stomach is full, which helps us eat less.

   DOES HIGH FIBER MAKE A DIFFERENCE?

   Researchers at the University of Minnesota found that eating whole grain, high-fiber barley for breakfast significantly decreased hunger before lunch, while eating whole wheat and refined rice foods did not.

3. **Fiber facilitates weight loss and maintenance.** Fiber moves fat through our digestive system faster so that absorption is significantly reduced.

4. **Fiber can reduce the risk of disease.** Soluble fiber helps lower blood cholesterol and glucose levels. This, in turn, reduces the risk of diabetes, high cholesterol, and heart disease.

5. **Fiber helps maintain regularity.** Fiber increases the movement of food through the digestive system. While it increases bulk (weight and size), it is also a natural stool softener, which facilitates bowel movement. As a result, fiber promotes regularity and helps avoid or eliminate constipation, hard stools, abdominal pain, and "sluggish bowel" syndrome.

WHAT ARE THE BEST SOURCES OF FIBER?

In its natural state—raw—fiber makes up a substantial part of whole fruit, whole vegetables, and whole grains. Many sources provide both soluble and insoluble fiber. For instance, the skins of fruit and root vegetables provide insoluble fiber, while the insides provide soluble fiber. Because soluble and insoluble fiber help the body to function in different ways, it is important to incorporate both types into meals and snacks.

EXAMPLES OF FIBER: SOLUBLE AND INSOLUBLE

SOLUBLE FIBER		
Artichokes	Broccoli	Peas
Barley	Flaxseed	Psyllium
Beans	Fruit	Root Vegetables
Berries	Oats	*(Insides)*
INSOLUBLE FIBER		
Corn Bran	Seeds	Wheat Bran
Fruit Skins	Vegetables	Whole Grain Foods
Lignans	Vegetable Skins	Whole Wheat Flour
	Nuts	

HOW SHOULD I INCORPORATE FIBER INTO MY DIET?

Simply put, the more *whole* vegetables, *whole* fruit, and *whole* grains that you eat, the better. Notice the key word: WHOLE. All three types of naturally fibrous foods lose fiber content when processed. For instance, foods made from white flour, e.g., bleached, refined, enriched, or unbleached—including pasta, pizza, and many breads and cereals—are poor sources of fiber even though they are made from wheat. As a result, focus on veggies, fruit, and grains in their most natural, least processed form. Here are ways to incorporate fiber into your day:

Did You Know?
The average American consumes only 5 to 10 grams of fiber a day. This is 15 to 20 grams LESS than what the FDA recommends.

- **Fruit.** Eat whole fruit whenever possible, and avoid bottled juices or those made from concentrate. Even 100 percent fruit juice and juices that contain pulp tend to lack fiber content. Aim to include at least two or three servings of whole fruit daily, preferably at breakfast and as part of a late-morning or midday snack.

- **Vegetables.** Eat vegetables as often and as much as possible. Aim to get a minimum of five to seven servings a day. Refer to chapter 7, *"Practice Makes Perfect,"* for portion sizes.
    - o **Lunch and dinner**. Incorporate veggies into both lunch and dinner menus to get a healthy "dose" in your diet. Eat a big, colorful salad for lunch. For dinner, always have a salad to start the meal plus another vegetable with the main course.
    - o **Mix it up!** Consume as many colors and kinds of vegetables as possible. This ensures maximum delivery of vitamins, minerals, and disease-fighting phytonutrients through food, rather than relying on supplements. Also, deep-colored veggies are richer in nutrients than their lighter counterparts. High-nutrient vegetables include broccoli, red peppers, orange peppers, tomatoes, dark, leafy greens (such as spinach), mixed greens, carrots, red cabbage,

eggplant, and zucchini. Also, vegetables in the lily family—asparagus, chives, onions, garlic, leeks, and shallots—have many sulfur-containing compounds that may fight cancer.

o **Limit starchy veggies.** Although starchy vegetables such as corn, peas, and potatoes are good for you, eat them in moderation. They tend to be higher in calories as compared to fibrous vegetables. The vegetables listed in the above paragraph—"*Mix it up!*"—are good examples of fibrous vegetables.

o **Go crazy with fibrous veggies.** You can NEVER eat too many fibrous veggies. So eat a LOT of them. Fibrous veggies are very low in calories, have virtually no fat, and boast tons of vital nutrients, all of which are critical to your health.

- **Whole Grains.** Whole grains tend to be higher in calories than vegetables or even fruit, so consume them in moderation. Always look for the "Whole Grain Stamp" and read the ingredient list on products to be sure they really contain fiber.

ADD FIBER SLOWLY!!

Adding more fiber to your diet will help you lose unwanted pounds and improve overall health! Include fiber gradually, however: too rapid an increase in consumption may result in flatulence and/or diarrhea. So take it slow until your body adjusts. Also, since fiber absorbs water, stay well hydrated and drink ample fluids.

- **Prepackaged Snacks.** If you're on the run and need to grab a quick prepackaged snack, strive for a ratio of 2 grams of fiber per 100 calories. Better yet, opt for those high in fiber and low in saturated fat. Some great snack bars that fill the bill and include high amounts of fiber are Gnu Flavor & Fiber, Kashi Go Lean, and Odwalla bars.

THE ONE-MINUTE SUMMARY

1. Incorporate high-fiber foods in every meal and snack.
2. Carbohydrates contain dietary fiber, which includes all parts of plant foods that your body can't absorb.
3. Fiber is important to your diet because it:
   - fills you up so you eat less;
   - stabilizes your energy and sugar levels;
   - facilitates weight loss and maintenance;
   - reduces risk of certain diseases;
   - maintains regularity in the digestive tract.
4. Fiber is found in whole vegetables, whole fruit, and whole grains. Because these have different types of fiber (insoluble and soluble), it is important to integrate all three into your diet.

3

PACK LEAN PROTEINS INTO EVERY MEAL

Whether you're a vegetarian, a carnivore, a vegan, or any other type of eater, it is imperative to incorporate lean proteins into your meals and snacks.

WHAT IS LEAN PROTEIN?

Proteins are nutrients that come from plants and animals. They are made up of amino acids, which are critical to life. Proteins are crucial to the structure of our bones, our skin, our hair and nails, our muscles, our blood, and our organs. *Lean* proteins, specifically, are those that are low in saturated fat. Saturated fat is known to raise LDL, the bad type of cholesterol, and, therefore, increase the risk of heart disease. LDL is referred to as bad cholesterol because, when oxidized, these particles can lead to artery-blocking blood clots. In contrast, HDL particles—the good cholesterol—sponge up excess cholesterol and carry it off for disposal. As a result, it is best to eat the leanest types of protein available to minimize LDL levels.

PROTEIN AND WEIGHT LOSS

In obese adults, a moderate-protein diet produces sustained weight loss and long-term changes in body composition and blood lipids. Researchers at the University of Illinois found that by increasing protein intake, subjects experienced increases in fat loss while increasing lean muscle tissue.

WHY ARE LEAN PROTEINS IMPORTANT?

1. **Lean proteins boost and maintain a healthy metabolism.** They build and preserve muscle mass, which underscores peak metabolic performance. Muscle mass burns more calories than fat: the more muscle, the faster the metabolism. Further, it is more difficult for the body to metabolize protein, so more calories are burned during digestion.

2. **Lean proteins are filling and satisfying.** Protein fills you up faster than a meal or snack made up primarily of carbohydrates and fat. Consequently, you eat less. Also, because it takes more time to digest, you feel fuller longer, diminishing hunger pangs between meals.

3. **Lean proteins are necessary for proper body function.** They not only transport nutrients throughout the body, they help generate essential hormones and enzymes the body requires to function properly.

4. **Lean proteins help prevent aging.** Proteins function as building blocks for bones, muscles, cartilage, skin, blood, enzymes, and hormones. As we age, proteins are important to maintain the structure of our hair and blood, preserve lean muscle mass, and assist growth. Protein is also an absolute necessity for healthy, beautiful, and youthful skin.

5. **Lean proteins help to ward off sickness.** Proteins repair and rebuild tissue and cells, and they support the immune system. Consequently, they help to ward off colds and other illnesses.

6. **Lean proteins provide energy.** Protein-rich foods increase brain levels of the amino acid tyrosine. Tyrosine is a key building block for the energizing neurochemicals dopamine and norepinephrine. As a result, protein can increase energy and make you feel more alert.

WHAT ARE THE BEST SOURCES OF LEAN PROTEIN?

Lean proteins are found in animals as well as plants and fall into two categories: complete and incomplete.

EXAMPLES OF LEAN PROTEIN

COMPLETE		
Chicken *(White Meat)*		Meat *(Lean Cuts)*
Dairy *(Non- and Low-fat)*		Quinoa
Egg Whites		Soy
Fish		Whey
INCOMPLETE		
Beans	Legumes	Seeds*
Grains	Nuts*	Vegetables

* Seeds and nuts are high in healthy fat and should be consumed in moderation. See chapter 4—"Enjoy Healthy Fats"—for more information.

- **Complete Proteins.** These contain all of the necessary amino acids required by the body. They are sufficient by themselves as a protein source and are found in quinoa, soy, and all animal proteins.

HIGH PROTEIN DIETS AND YOUR HEALTH

Cutting out any nutrient from your diet is unhealthy and may be detrimental to your health. Fad diets often remove critical nutrients in favor of others, e.g., carbohydrates in favor of proteins and fats, fats in favor of high carbs, etc. The key to success is to balance carbohydrates with proteins. Further, reducing highly processed carbohydrates while increasing lean protein and complex, unrefined carbohydrates will improve levels of blood triglycerides and HDL. These, in turn, reduce the risk of heart attack, stroke, and other cardiovascular diseases.

- **Incomplete Proteins.** These are found in plants and don't contain all the necessary amino acids your body needs. On their own, they are not sufficient as protein sources.

HOW SHOULD I INCORPORATE LEAN PROTEINS INTO MY DIET?

Try to include them with every snack and meal. You can have a complete protein independently or combine different incomplete proteins to create a complete one. Avoid, however, consuming a diet that is too high in proteins. Fad diets have been shown to be detrimental to your health. A good rule of thumb: lean proteins should make up 20 to 40 percent of daily caloric intake. This equates to an average of 5 to 8 grams of protein per 100 calories.

COMPLETE PROTEINS

- **Meat and Poultry.** Opt for fresh meat and chicken whenever possible. Choose the leanest cuts of red meat and only white meat poultry. Avoid deli meats that are high in sodium. If you do purchase deli meats, read the labels and check for sodium and/or MSG content. Additionally,

CALCIUM AND DAIRY

Although you may not be lactose intolerant, dairy may still have an effect on you. Many people suffer from bloating, gassiness, and indigestion from consuming dairy products, and when they cut back on or eliminate dairy from their diet, many, if not all, of these symptoms disappear. If you are one of these individuals or dislike dairy altogether, you can get calcium from other sources, such as dark green, leafy vegetables and broccoli. Both are also good sources of vitamin K, which is another key nutrient for bone health.

avoid packaged or processed meats that contain fillers, additives, and preservatives. Grill or broil red meats, and bake or grill poultry. Avoid heavy sautéing or frying.

- **Dairy.** Dairy foods, such as milk, yogurt, and cheese, can be good protein sources. Opt for 1 percent milk or non-fat dairy products; 2 percent, whole milk, and, of course, cream are high in saturated fat. Also, whey protein powders are a substantial source of complete lean protein. Use them in fruit smoothies to create a well-balanced meal or snack.

- **Eggs.** Eggs are an excellent source of protein. Egg yolks, however, are high in cholesterol, which can cause potential health risks. If you have high cholesterol or if it runs in your family, stick to eating egg whites.

Did You Know?

Although often called the "supergrain," quinoa (pronounced keen-wah) is a seed related to the spinach family.

- **Fish.** Eat fish grilled, baked, or poached. Sushi is also a great option; however, choose brown over white rice when possible, since brown rice has more fiber.

- **Quinoa.** Quinoa is one of the most complete foods found in nature because it contains protein, enzymes, vitamins and minerals, fiber, antioxidants, and phytonutrients. Additionally, it is gluten-free, which makes it a great source of fiber for those who have gluten allergies.

- **Soy.** Soy is a legume and is one of only two plant-based proteins that are complete. Although soy is a better choice than red meat, it's still best to consume it in moderation (two to four servings per week).

INCOMPLETE PROTEINS

Other than soy and quinoa, plant proteins do not have all the essential amino acids required by the body. If you are a vegetarian, it is important to have a variety of *in-complete proteins* to ensure you get the *complete protein* needed in your diet.

PAIRING INCOMPLETE PROTEINS

To get complete proteins from incomplete sources, combine a protein from the *Grains* category with a protein in the *Legumes, Nuts/Seeds*, or *Vegetables* categories. Popular combinations include brown rice and beans, oatmeal and nuts, peanut butter and whole grain bread, or tofu and brown rice. If you don't combine these at each meal, make sure to do so at least through the day.

GRAINS

Barley	Bulgur	Rye
Brown Rice	Cornmeal	Wheat
Buckwheat	Oats	Whole Grain Pasta

LEGUMES	NUTS/SEEDS*	VEGETABLES**
Beans	Cashews	Asparagus
Chickpeas	Pumpkin Seeds	Broccoli
Dried Peas	Sesame Seeds	Cauliflower
Lentils	Sunflower Seeds	Potatoes
Peanuts	Walnuts	
	Other Nuts	

* *Nuts are high in fat, so it is best to eat them in moderation. Refer to recommended serving sizes in chapter 7, "Practice Makes Perfect."*

** *Legumes, nuts, and seeds tend to be higher in protein than vegetables. High-protein vegetable sources include asparagus, broccoli, cauliflower, and potatoes.*

THE ONE-MINUTE SUMMARY

1. Incorporate lean proteins with every meal and snack.
2. Proteins are nutrients crucial to the structure of the body. Specifically, lean proteins are those that are low in saturated fat.
3. Lean proteins are important to a healthy diet because they:
   - boost and maintain a healthy metabolism;
   - kill hunger pangs and satisfy the appetite for longer periods of time;
   - are important to healthy bodily function;
   - keep us looking young.
4. Complete lean proteins come from meats, poultry, fish, dairy, quinoa, or soy. Incomplete lean proteins come from grains, legumes, nuts, seeds, and vegetables.
5. Consume an average of 5 to 8 grams of protein per 100 calories.

4

ENJOY HEALTHY FATS

Good news: "Fat is good for you!" In fact, a healthy diet requires fat. Unquestionably, some—specifically saturated and trans fats—have earned a disastrous reputation. Justifiably so! They raise LDL (the bad type of cholesterol) and vastly increase the risk of heart disease. Saturated fats are found in fatty meats and fatty dairy products; trans fats, which are mostly industrially created, are found in fried foods. There are healthy fats, however, that are essential to your health and, consequently, vital to a healthy diet.

WHAT ARE HEALTHY FATS?

Healthy fats include monounsaturated and polyunsaturated fats, especially omega-3 essential fatty acids (EFAs). Omega-3s are a special type of polyunsaturated fat that are absolutely necessary to our well-being. Unfortunately, our bodies cannot produce them on our own and, as a result, we depend on food and supplements to get them.

OMEGA-6 ESSENTIAL FATTY ACIDS

You may have heard of omega-6 essential fatty acids (EFAs). Omega-6 EFAs are most commonly found in vegetable oils, including corn, safflower, sesame, sunflower, and soybean oils. They can also be found in borage oil, evening primrose oil, hemp oil, walnut oil, and wheat germ.

Although omega-6 EFAs provide health benefits, the consumption ratio of omega-6s to omega-3s is critically important. The ratio of omega-6 to omega-3 should be no more than 4:1, with an optimal ratio of 1:1. Consumption ratios greater than 4:1 have been linked to long-term diseases such as asthma, depression, heart disease, arthritis, and cancer.

With vegetable oils so prominent in packaged foods, fast foods, and restaurant cuisine, Americans get their fair share of omega-6s. As a result, most Americans tend to overconsume omega-6 EFAs, while they underconsume omega-3s. As a matter of fact, the average consumption ratio among Americans is approximately 6:1.

Since the American diet appears to lack sufficient omega-3s, we need to focus on the importance of including them in the proper ratio.

WHY ARE HEALTHY FATS IMPORTANT?

Although each type of healthy fat provides its own specific benefits, the following are common to all.

1. **Healthy fats support essential body function.** Healthy fats improve blood cholesterol levels, ease inflammation, and sta-

bilize heart rhythms. They lubricate joints and assist in the manufacture of hormones. Without them, hormone production drops, and normal chemical reactions are interrupted, potentially causing weight gain, decreased reproductive capability, and other health issues.

2. **Healthy fats are needed to absorb fat-soluble vitamins.** Vitamins A, D, E, and K are important to healthy vision, skin, and teeth. As fat-soluble vitamins, they are absorbed through the intestinal tract with the help of fats. These vitamins are essential for our bodies to stay healthy, including cell differentiation, immune system function, and bone strength.

3. **Healthy fats boost metabolism.** They aid in the production of testosterone, instrumental in building and maintaining lean muscle mass. As previously discussed in chapter 3, *"Pack Lean Proteins into Every Meal,"* lean muscle mass boosts metabolism because muscle burns more calories than fat.

4. **Healthy fats help to protect against disease.** Because healthy fats lower cholesterol and diminish the formation of blood clots, they help decrease the risk of heart disease. Further, they boost immune-system function, maintain bone health, and work to prevent inflammation in blood vessels, which lowers the potential risk of autoimmune diseases, such as rheumatoid arthritis.

5. **Healthy fats promote healthy skin.** Skin is made up of fats and proteins. Healthy fats manufacture and repair cell membranes, stimulate skin and hair growth, and support the tone, texture, and resilience of skin. Omega-3s, specifically, create the oil barrier that protects the skin as well as the body against fluid loss and infection.

OIL PROCESSING: NUTRITIONAL IMPACT

Oils are not all created equal. Specifically, some are more refined than others. Many oils are produced by using heat, alone or with the chemical hexane. Heat can degrade the flavor, nutritional value, and color of the oil, while hexane, in large quantities, may be dangerous to our health.

Unrefined oils, however, are richer in nutrients, more robust, and true to their natural flavors. Expeller pressing is a chemical-free process that extracts oil from nuts or seeds by crushing them at various temperatures. Cold expeller-pressed oil, specifically, is done at very low heat—no higher than 120°F. Generally, harder nuts require higher temperatures. And although the expeller-pressed oils are not treated with hexane during the expeller-pressing process, they may be treated with hexane afterwards to extract more of the remaining oil.

When you shop for oils, look for those that are unrefined, cold expeller-pressed to ensure you are getting the highest quality oil.

WHAT ARE THE BEST SOURCES OF HEALTHY FATS?

Healthy fats can be found in nuts, certain oils, fish, seeds, and vegetables. The following table provides a list of the best food sources for monounsaturated and polyunsaturated fats as well as omega-3 essential fatty acids.

SOURCES OF HEALTHY FATS

POLYUNSATURATED AND OMEGA-3 FATS*		
Cod	Flaxseeds	Halibut
Dried Cloves	Mustard Seeds	Salmon
Dried Oregano		Walnuts
MONOUNSATURATED FATS		
Almonds	Hazelnuts	Peanuts
Avocados	Olives	Peanut Butter
Canola Oil	Olive Oil	Sesame Seeds
Cashews		Tahini Paste

* *Omega-6 essential fatty acids are not included in this table because we get enough omega-6 fats in our diet naturally. Refer to the insert on omega-6 fats earlier on page 36.*

WHAT FOODS SHOULD I AVOID?

Avoid foods that are high in saturated fats or those that contain trans fats. The most common unhealthy fatty foods include:

- **Fatty Red Meat and Poultry Skin.** Red meat and poultry skin contain saturated fat. Further, meats that are processed or come from fatty parts of the animal are especially unhealthy. These include bacon, sausage, hot dogs, salami, and chopped meat. The leanest cuts of meat are those that include the word "round" or "loin" in their name—for example, top sirloin, top round, and tenderloin. The leanest cuts of poultry are white meat parts.

- **Whole Fat Dairy.** Made with whole milk or cream and high in saturated fat, these include butter, cream, yogurt, half-and-half, whole milk, and ice cream. Because dairy products can provide a variety of health benefits, consume those made from whole milk sparingly and stick to low-fat options on a regular basis. A good rule of thumb is to have whole milk products no more than once a week.

- **Fried Foods.** These are loaded with saturated fat. Worse yet, fried foods prepared in restaurants and fast food venues usually pack a whopping amount of trans fats.

- **Commercially Prepared and Baked Goods.** Commercially prepared foods, as we discussed previously, include a lot of unhealthy ingredients. Furthermore, they are heavily processed and deliver an extraordinary amount of empty calories.

- **Fast Foods.** These represent tasty fare for many but are loaded with both saturated and trans fats. The best thing to do is avoid fast food restaurants completely.

HOW SHOULD I INCORPORATE HEALTHY FATS INTO MY DIET?

Even with the healthiest of fats, it is important to remember a little goes a long way. Healthy fats are still high in calories and, if eaten in excess, can contribute mightily to weight gain: consume them SPARINGLY. A good rule of thumb: healthy fats should make up 20 to 30 percent of your daily caloric intake. This equates to an average of 2½ to 3 grams of fat per 100 calories.

- **When Cooking.** Olive oil and canola oil are great for cooking. Use extra-virgin olive oil (EVOO): it provides significant health benefits over ordinary olive oil. Olive oils that are not extra-virgin tend to be processed or mixed with other types of oils, thereby diminishing their quality. Also, look for olive oil and canola oil cooking sprays in your grocery store. They are healthier than other cooking sprays. A great product, easily available, is

Misto, a refillable oil or dressing spray applicator. It allows you to use less oil by moderating the amount used. Use it for all of your cooking oils. Also, pay attention to the level of heat you use for your various oils (refer to the "Smoke Points and Cooking" chart on the next page).

- **When Baking.** Olive oil isn't always preferred for baking: some people don't like the taste. Instead, use canola oil in lieu of traditional corn or vegetable oil. The flavor is not as strong, but it still is a good source of monounsaturated fat.

- **Something Smells Fishy.** Fatty fish, such as salmon, halibut, and cod, are excellent in providing omega-3s. Although it's preferable to obtain nutrients directly from food sources, if you don't like fish, fish oil supplements are a viable option.

- **When Entertaining.** Olives are a great source of monounsaturated fats. Serve olives, olive tapenade, and bruschetta drizzled with olive oil. Additionally, homemade guacamole made with fresh avocado (a seriously healthy fruit) is easy to prepare and a delicious crowd pleaser.

- **As Snacks.** Some of the best snacks are nuts. Walnuts and almonds, especially, are full of healthy fats. A healthy serving size is approximately one-quarter cup of shelled, unsalted nuts. Further, they are easy to take with you on the go!

- **In Salads.** Nuts, avocados, and olives are all delicious in salads and offer fabulous, healthy fats. When preparing dressings, stay with olive oil, lemon juice, and vinegars. Avoid bottled salad dressings: they tend to have substantial amounts of unhealthy ingredients. Also, don't overload healthy fats into your salad. Choose one serving of fat per salad so that you don't turn your salad into an unhealthy dish (refer to chapter 10, *"Recipes,"* for some ideas).

SMOKE POINTS AND COOKING

Each type of oil has a "smoke point," which is the specific temperature at which the oil starts to break down, its molecular structure begins to change, and it can become unhealthy. The higher the smoke point, the higher the temperature the oil can withstand. As a result, each type of oil should be used for the cooking method that is most appropriate to its individual smoke point and heat tolerance.

Smoke Point	Oil*	Best Use
225°F	Flaxseed (UR)	Salads
320°F	Corn (UR)	Baking (low heat) Light Sautéing Pressure Cooking Salads
320°F	Extra-Virgin Olive Oil (UR)	
320°F	Peanut (UR)	
320°F	Walnut (UR)	
350°F	Sesame (UR)	
390°F	Macadamia Nut (UR)	Baking (medium heat) Sautéing Stir-frying
400°F	Canola (R)	
450°F	Coconut (R)	
450°F	Safflower (R)	
450°F	Soybean/Soy (R)	Deep Browning Deep-frying Searing
450°F	Sunflower (R)	
520°F	Avocado (R)	

* Unrefined oils (UR) have lower smoke points than refined (R) or semirefined oils. Refined oils, however, tend to lose some flavor, nutrients, and color in the refining process.

- **In Shakes and Yogurt Parfaits.** Milled (or ground) flaxseed has a delightful, nutty flavor and is filled with healthy omega-3 fats and fiber. A couple of tablespoons in cereal, shakes, or yogurt parfaits provide an extra healthy kick.

- **Keep Them in Balance.** Balance out your fats. It makes sense to have one "fat food" in each meal or snack, but any more can produce an unbalanced diet. For instance, if you traditionally have cereal and milk in the morning for breakfast, use nonfat milk and a healthy fatty cereal, such as Kashi, to get in your dose of monounsaturated and/or polyunsaturated fats. If for lunch you have sandwiches, opt for only one fat—such as cheese, avocado, or hummus—NOT two or three.

THE ONE-MINUTE SUMMARY

1. Healthy fats are important to a healthy diet.
2. Healthy fats include monounsaturated and polyunsaturated types, specifically, omega-3 essential fatty acids (EFAs).
3. Common benefits of healthy fats include:
   - support of bodily functions, the lubrication of joints, and the manufacture of important hormones;
   - stabilization of a healthy metabolism;
   - disease prevention;
   - beautiful, healthy, youthful skin.
4. Nuts, olive and canola oils, flaxseed, and fatty fish are some of the best sources of healthy fats.
5. When incorporating healthy fats into your diet, use them sparingly: they are still high in fat and calories!
6. Have an average of 2½ to 3 grams of fat per 100 calories.

EAT SMALL, OFTEN, AND MINDFULLY

Overeating, undereating, and skipping meals are all-too-common behaviors. Unfortunately, these habits can mess up your metabolism, leave you ravenously hungry, or make you feel uncomfortably "stuffed." Truth be told, portion control doesn't necessarily require counting calories, which can be tedious at best. To ensure you are eating correctly, commit to eating mindfully and consuming small meals throughout the day.

WHAT DOES "SMALL, OFTEN, AND MINDFUL EATING" MEAN?

The "small" and "often" parts of this statement are easy: five to six times a day, every two to three hours. "Mindful" is far more challenging. Mindful eating requires you to tune in to how you feel—mentally, emotionally, and physically—before, during, and after you eat.

WHY IS EATING SMALL, OFTEN, AND MINDFULLY IMPORTANT?

1. **It helps control your appetite.** If you allow yourself to get extremely hungry between meals, you run the risk of overeating when you do eat. By consuming small meals at regular intervals, you don't have time to get tremendously hungry.

Result: better appetite control. Eating mindfully allows you to identify and deal with reactive, habitual patterns of thinking, feeling, and acting in relationship to food.

2. **It keeps energy levels stable.** When you eat regularly, you constantly provide your body with the nutrients and energy it needs to function productively. Additionally, sugar levels are stabilized, which helps to keep you active and alert throughout the day.

3. **It bolsters metabolism.** Because your body requires energy to digest, absorb, and metabolize food, you burn more calories when you eat than when you don't. As a result, the more often you eat, the greater the caloric burn. Conversely, when you eat less frequently, your metabolism slows down to compensate, and if you go too long between meals, your body thinks it's in "starvation mode," causing your metabolism to shut down even further.

4. **It bolsters awareness of your relationship with food.** Many of us find ourselves eating when we are stressed, depressed, bored, or just because food is in front of us—even when we aren't really hungry. This can sabotage our attempt to eat healthy. Eating mindfully makes us aware of our eating habits so that we can address those in particular that are tied to emotional needs.

HOW DO I PRACTICE SMALL, OFTEN, AND MINDFUL EATING?

Eating small, regular meals and being mindful through the process requires both planning and practice. Like any other habit, however, repetition will produce a natural integration into your lifestyle.

- **Never Skip Breakfast.** Daily breakfast is important to eating healthy. As a matter of fact, those who consistently eat a healthy breakfast tend to weigh less than those who don't. Breakfast helps stabilize blood sugar and hormone levels while revving the metabolism to burn more calories through the course of the day.

BOTTOMLESS BOWLS AND ENDLESS BUFFETS!

Many eaters rely on visual cues, such as an empty plate, to decide when to stop eating. But what if the plate was never clean or the bowl never empty? To test this question, Cornell University researcher Dr. Brian Wansink created a bottomless soup bowl, which secretly refilled during a meal. He found that diners eating from the refillable bowl ate 73 percent more soup than diners who ate from a normal bowl.

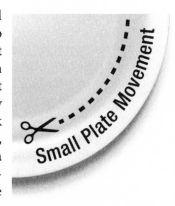

SIZE MATTERS

Wansink found that plate size matters. By reducing plate diameter from 12 to 10 inches, people ate 22 percent fewer calories. Consider joining the Small Plate Challenge, which asks consumers to use a 10-inch plate for their biggest meals.

Photo courtesy of http://www.smallplatemovement.org

- **Downsize Your Main Meals.** Instead of three large meals a day—breakfast, lunch, and dinner—decrease portion sizes and allocate some of the food for snacks. You will spread what would normally be three meals into five. Here's a good schedule to try:

    Breakfast: 7:30 a.m. to 8:30 a.m.
    Morning Snack: 10:00 a.m. to 11:00 a.m.
    Lunch: 12:30 p.m. to 1:30 p.m.
    Afternoon Snack: 3:00 p.m. to 4:00 p.m.
    Dinner: 6:00 p.m. to 7:00 p.m.

    It is best to eat no later than 7:30 at night and to stay up for at least two hours after eating. A late meal can make it difficult to get a good night's sleep.

- **Snack.** This may sound unhealthy, but in reality, it is quite the opposite. Snacking—with care and purpose—can be both healthy and satisfying. Prepare ahead so that you have tasty, filling, and healthy snacks with you. Check the recipe section for ideas.

- **Pre-plate Your Food.** Cornell University Food and Brand Lab researchers found that individuals who pre-plated their food ate approximately 14 percent less than those who took smaller amounts and returned for seconds and thirds. Pre-plate your meals or snacks before you start eating so that you have a visual stopping point. Avoid eating chips straight out of the bag or ice cream from the carton.

- **Turn Off the TV.** Make mealtime its own time. Turn off the TV, close the magazine, and put down your book while eating. These types of distractions can lead to longer mealtimes and less careful consumption monitoring.

Research has shown that both children and adults snack more when watching TV. A controlled study found that the longer people watched TV, the more they ate. Participants who watched TV for an hour ate 28 percent more popcorn than if they watched for a half hour.

- **Be Last.** Research has shown that when we dine with others, we tend to sit at meals longer and, as a result, eat more. On average, if you eat with one other person, you'll eat 35 percent more than you would have alone. If you eat with a group of seven or more, you'll eat nearly twice as much food as you would alone. This is partially due to the fact that when food remains on the table, our visual "hunger" cues persist. If you eat with a group, be last to start eating. Waiting will create less downtime to think about or want food.

- **Plan Well.** We all get busy and, inevitably, don't have time to prepare a meal or snack. It pays to plan for such occasions. Remember, skipped meals will slow down metabolism and produce extra hunger. When this happens, you eat more than you want or need. If you know your schedule will be tight, pack snacks to take off the edge: try a nutrition bar, or a piece of fruit coupled with a quarter-cup of nuts.

- **Evaluate Your Environment.** Keep your healthiest whole foods front and center. The less that unhealthy foods are in your face, the less likely you will be tempted to eat them. For instance, if you typically keep a bowl of candy on the coffee table or kitchen counter, swap it for a bowl of cherries. If your fridge or cabinets are loaded with unhealthy snacks, put them toward the back and bring the healthiest foods to the forefront.

VARIETY AND DIET

Researchers from Brown University Medical School believe that eating a monotonous diet can promote weight loss. In a study published in 2006, they found that subjects in a reduced-variety condition decreased their weekly intake of calories from snack foods by 63 percent.

Reducing variety in your diet may help you to eat less. The key is to do it in a way that doesn't make you feel deprived. For example, you could eat the same healthy lunch every day, but vary the vegetables that you include in the meal.

- **Be Simple and Repetitive.** Research shows the more varied our diet, the more likely we are to eat greater quantities and to increase our intake of unhealthy foods. Keep things simple and a bit repetitive: it will help you eat less and be more aware of tendencies to splurge or veer from the five principles. Find several very healthy breakfasts, lunches, and/or snacks that can be your go-to meals. Refer to chapter 10, *"Recipes,"* for some ideas.

- **Journal.** Keep a journal to document how you feel physically and mentally—before, during, and after meals and snacks. You should pay attention to:

  1. **Appetite.** Evaluate your appetite on a scale of 0 to 5: 0 represents "extremely hungry," 5 "extremely full." Whenever possible, strive never to be a 0 or a 5. If hunger sets in, aim for a rating no lower than 1; after you have eaten, you shouldn't be fuller than a 4.

2. **Emotional Status.** When eating, tune in to your emotional state. Are you stressed? Depressed? Happy? Relaxed? Bored? Note your feelings in order to understand what triggers your eating. Are you really hungry? Are you using food to fill an empty void? Is food an automatic go-to when celebrating? Noting these feelings will help you distinguish between real hunger and emotional hunger.

3. **What You Eat.** Document what and how much you eat. This will help you identify those foods that are most gratifying and filling as they apply to actual hunger as well as emotional triggers. It will also enable you to determine how balanced your snacks and meals are.

Did You Know?

Eating slowly can help you lose weight and eat less: it takes twenty minutes for your brain to know you've eaten enough. So slow down and enjoy!

THE ONE-MINUTE SUMMARY

1. To ensure you eat just enough, eat mindfully and eat small meals throughout the day.
2. Consume small meals or snacks five to six times a day, every two to three hours; be sure to tune in to how you feel mentally, emotionally, and physically—before, during, and after you eat.
3. Enjoying small meals often and staying mindful of how you eat will help you to:
   - control your appetite;
   - keep your energy levels stable;
   - boost your metabolism;
   - be aware of your relationship with food.
4. To best incorporate this principle into your lifestyle, plan ahead so that you can avoid extreme hunger and never have to skip a meal or snack.

PART 2

THE "GET REAL" TOOLKIT

INTRODUCTION

After reading Part 1, you should have a solid understanding of the "GET REAL" principles and approach to eating healthy for life. In Part 2, you'll receive the tools necessary to effectively implement them into your day-to-day lifestyle to look and feel your best—today, tomorrow, and always.

1. **The Plate and Beyond.** Learn five helpful tips that will facilitate eating healthy, plus five additional tips that will take you "beyond the plate." These will further enhance your efforts to achieve established goals.

2. **Practice Makes Perfect.** Don't obsess over calories. Instead, learn what foods should be on your grocery list, appropriate portion sizes, and healthy ingredients that can substitute for less healthy choices when baking or cooking.

3. **Preferred Brands.** There may be times when you'll have to resort to packaged goods. Refer to this handy list for brands that are preferred: they'll significantly facilitate meal planning and preparation.

4. **It's All in the Label.** When attempting to decipher labels on food products, you need to know exactly what the nutrition labels are stating. This chapter provides the tools to understand what the product provides, enabling you to make smart decisions.

5. **Recipes.** And perhaps the best piece of the pie: forty delicious recipes that put the "GET REAL" principles to the taste test!

Part 2 is your toolkit to turn the five "GET REAL" principles into REALITY. Before you begin the journey toward a diet-free lifestyle, it's important to acquire the proper mind-set.

1. **Make This Your Choice.** Continually remind yourself that eating healthy is a choice—something you want to do—and a lifestyle, not "dieting." To truly be successful, you have to *want* this, not feel forced into it.

2. **Small Change for Big Impact.** Attempting to make major changes all at once can be overwhelming. Instead, set one or two smaller, more manageable goals each week. When you have successfully accomplished these, move on to other more realistic goals. For instance, if you consume a lot of sugar, focus on cutting back for a few weeks until you've made definite progress. Then decide on another change, such as cutting back on red meat or other fattier proteins. Small changes, consistently applied, will have a big positive impact in the long run.

3. **Change Takes Time.** Change does not happen overnight. As you embark on a healthier lifestyle, realize that change takes time and allow an adequate timeline to ensure success.

4. **Stay Positive.** Shut out negative thoughts that can sabotage the best intentions. Instead, continually remind yourself of all the *positives* that will result from a healthier lifestyle: feeling good, looking great, and preventing the onset of disease and illness.

5. **Enjoy the Process.** As you discover quality foods, concentrate on how delicious they taste. Acknowledge and be aware of the satisfaction you get from food that is naturally filling and nutritious—and even better, flavors that are real instead of artificial.

6

THE PLATE AND BEYOND

The five "GET REAL" principles are your foundation for eating well and feeling great. The following tips should be helpful as you implement them and integrate them into your lifestyle.

THE PLATE

1. **85%/15% Rule.** While eating healthy is important, there are those times when we all wish to indulge a little. The 85%/15% rule of thumb is perfect for such occasions. This means that 85 percent of the time, or six out of seven days a week, you follow the five "GET REAL" principles; one day of the week, whatever day you choose, you give yourself permission to fall off the wagon. For instance, if you have a special event on a Saturday evening, maintain the five principles Sunday through Friday and let loose on Saturday. You'll feel less guilty and enjoy yourself thoroughly. Further, depriving yourself will not be sustainable for the long term. If you are strongly craving a piece of cheesecake, allow yourself a bite or two—not the whole piece—and be sure the indulgence doesn't become a daily occurrence. By giving in to your cravings once in a while, it will be easier to stay on track the majority of the time.

2. **Sugar and Artificial Sweeteners.** This tip is an extension of principle #1, *"Keep It Whole, Keep It Natural, Keep It Simple."*

CAN YOU RETRAIN YOUR TASTE BUDS?

Many people report that cravings for junk foods subside after they transition from an unhealthy diet of processed foods to a healthier diet of whole foods. If you eat a healthy diet, your insulin, leptin, and blood sugar levels should be balanced. With this balance, your body will crave sugar less often.

Diminish your intake of processed sugars and artificial sweeteners, including table sugar, confectioners' sugar, brown sugar, aspartame, sucralose, Sugar In The Raw, Splenda, NutraSweet, Sweet'n Low, and Equal. In addition, aim to weed out foods that have added sugars in them. This can include those mentioned above as well as corn syrups and high-fructose corn syrups. This may require some time, but here are a few suggestions.

- **Coffee and Tea.** If you drink coffee or tea, try to cut back, little by little, on the sugar you use each week. In lieu of sugar or artificial sweeteners, try low-fat or skim milk: they have their own natural sugars.

- **Baked Goods.** Avoid store-bought baked goods. Store-bought cookies and cakes tend to be loaded with extra sugars, artificial ingredients, and preservatives. If you want to indulge, try making them yourself using healthier ingredients, such as whole-wheat and other whole-grain flours (healthy ingredient substitutions are covered in chapter 7, "*Practice Makes Perfect*").

- **Yogurts.** Instead of eating yogurt that is already sweetened, eat plain yogurt sweetened with fresh fruit (mash the fruit to release the natural sugars).

ALL YOGURTS AREN'T CREATED EQUAL

Compared with traditional yogurts, Greek yogurts are higher in protein and lower in sugar, so they make a wonderful ingredient for a well-balanced meal or snack. Greek yogurts are also creamier than their traditional counterparts, giving recipes a richer, more delicious taste. Some brands to try include Fage, Oikos by Stonyfield, and Chobani.

- **Sodas.** Instead of drinking soda, have a glass filled with three parts club soda and one part 100 percent fruit juice. Or consider club soda with a splash of lemon or lime.

3. **Hold the Salt but Not the Spice.** Salt (sodium) causes water retention and, often, a bloated feeling. Further, too much sodium can cause high blood pressure. Instead, use a variety of spices to keep your taste buds satisfied and happy while providing easy and simple dishes with a whole new flavor (see Simple Baked Chicken in chapter 10, *"Recipes"*). Spices are flavorful and essentially noncaloric. Some popular spices to try include garlic, curry, mustard seeds, cloves, capers, cilantro, pepper, and cinnamon.

4. **Eat In, Why Don't You?** Save restaurants for special occasions, as a treat, or as part of your 85%/15% rule. Dining out can lead a healthy diet astray. When cooking for yourself, however, you have full disclosure about all ingredients in the recipe. You know what is incorporated in every meal, without risking hidden, high-caloric ingredients, such as butter. You can also depend on the quality of ingredients used. At home, you can control the portion sizes and can avoid the temptation of unhealthy menu items. Last but not least, eating in can save a lot of money.

5. **Keep Things Simple.** The "GET REAL" principles are not difficult to put into action. Keeping things simple for a few weeks—or until you get the hang of your new way of eating—will make it easier. Some ideas:

   - **Big-Batch Cooking.** Cook big batches of a recipe on a Sunday night to last you through the week. This will make the "what to make for dinner" conundrum a no-brainer and free you to focus on breakfast, lunch, and snack decisions instead.

   - **Know What You Like.** Find healthy recipes you enjoy and rotate them during the course of several weeks (for some ideas, refer to chapter 10, "*Recipes*"). Planning and preparing these will help you stay on track and keep you from craving unhealthier foods.

   - **Clean Out Your Closets.** Every week, give away five foods in your pantry that don't follow the five principles. When you shop, don't buy foods that are on the "avoid" list or those that you know are unhealthy. This will not only help you ease into a new shopping mode, it will eliminate those foods detrimental to your new lifestyle.

BEYOND THE PLATE

1. **Strength Train and Exercise.** Living a healthy lifestyle isn't just about eating right. It also requires us to move our butts and incorporate activity into our daily regimens. Strength, cardio, and flexibility training are all important to keep bones and hearts strong, metabolisms high, and bodies free from injury. In order to stay motivated, find a variety of activities you enjoy, and get in one or more of those activities for approximately one hour at least three times a week. This should include two twenty- to thirty-minute sessions of strength training weekly. If you're not into weight lifting, you

can enjoy yoga and Pilates (both incorporate strength training) as well as other forms of exercise that require muscular strength, such as rowing, tennis, gymnastics, and others.

2. **Hydrate.** Stay well hydrated through the day, every day. Since our bodies are composed of approximately 65 percent water, they require substantial replenishment of H_2O to function properly. Proper hydration flushes toxins, ensures proper digestive and bodily functions, curbs hunger, and helps fight aging. When possible, drink water, unsweetened green tea, or club soda. If water doesn't appeal, add a wedge of lemon, sliced cucumber, or a splash of 100 percent fruit juice for flavor. To ensure you are receiving adequate water intake, divide your weight (in pounds) by two. The number you get equals the ounces of water you should drink each day. This formula gives you a guide that won't under- or overhydrate your body.*

Hydration Formula:

$$\frac{\text{weight in pounds}}{2} = \text{number of ounces}$$

Example of a 140-pound individual:

$$\frac{140 \text{ pounds}}{2} = 70 \text{ ounces}$$

* *This hydration formula doesn't work for people who are obese. As a result, if you are 50 percent to 100 percent above your ideal body weight, consult your physician on this subject.*

3. **Get Your Zs.** Adequate sleep is highly beneficial to your health as well as your waistline. Those who get seven to eight hours of sleep each night tend to weigh less than individuals who are sleep deprived. Try to go to bed at the same time every night and wake up at the same time every morning. Also,

promote sound sleep by avoiding caffeine after noon, eating at least two to three hours before bedtime, and limiting alcohol intake.

4. **Drink Moderately.** Alcohol adds a lot of empty calories to a healthy diet. As a matter of fact, it adds seven calories per gram of alcohol, as compared to nine calories per gram of fat and four calories per gram of protein and/or gram of carbohydrates. By the same token, alcohol, in moderation, can help raise your HDL, the good cholesterol. This is true no matter what type of alcohol you consume. Recent research suggests that the heart-health benefit of alcohol is increased if moderate consumption is consistent: three to seven times a week, as opposed to sporadic consumption. To balance the benefits and the calories, women should limit themselves to no more than one drink a day; men, no more than two. One drink is 4 ounces of wine, 12 ounces of beer (a bottle or can), or 1 ounce of hard liquor.

5. **Manage Stress.** Stress is part of life. Managing stress so it isn't overwhelming is critical in maintaining a healthy lifestyle. When we are overstressed, we find ways to soothe ourselves, and often we do so with food. Exercising, getting enough sleep, and spending downtime either alone or with loved ones are all ways to help diminish the impact of stress on our lives.

7

PRACTICE MAKES PERFECT

Planning your menus, shopping for groceries, and preparing meals are all important in developing healthy habits. In this chapter, you'll acquire the information necessary to make smart choices both at the grocery store and at home.

THE PERFECT GROCERY LIST

All of the following grocery lists are comprised of whole foods. Cooking and baking with these ingredients will ensure that you sustain a diet that is as whole and nutritious as possible. Furthermore, foods are grouped into categories so that any food within a group can be substituted for another in the same group. For instance, under Protein and Dairy, a 3-ounce chicken breast can be substituted for ½ cup of plain, nonfat Greek yogurt. Similarly, under the Grains and Starchy Carbohydrates category, ½ cup of beans can be substituted for ¼ cup of freshly made hummus.

Fibrous Vegetables: All fresh, fibrous vegetables are approved. Those listed below are some of the most nutritious. Look for in-season veggies to ensure the freshest quality. (Serving sizes are ½ cup nonleafy vegetables or 1 cup raw, leafy vegetables).

Artichoke Hearts	Cucumber	Red Cabbage
Arugula	Eggplant	Red Peppers
Asparagus	Green Beans	Spinach
Broccoli	Mixed Greens	Squash
Carrots	Onions	Tomatoes
Cauliflower		Zucchini

Fruit: All fresh fruit is approved. Here are some serving sizes for those that are most commonly eaten. Look for in-season fruit to ensure the freshest quality.

Apples (1 medium)	Mixed Berries (1 c. frozen)
Bananas (1 small or ½ large)	Oranges (1 medium)
Blueberries (1 c.)	Raspberries (1 c.)
Grapefruit (½ medium)	Strawberries (1 c.)
Kiwi (2 small)	Tangerines (2 small)

Grains and Starchy Carbohydrates

Barley (½ c.)	Old-fashioned Rolled Oats (½ c. cooked)
Beans—any variety (½ cup)	
Brown Rice (⅓ c. cooked)	Popping Corn—nonmicrowavable (3 c. cooked)
Bulgur (½ c. cooked)	
Corn (½ c. cooked)	Quinoa (½ c.)
Edamame (½ c. shelled)	Sweet Potatoes (½ c.)
Hummus (¼ c.)	Whole-Grain Pasta (½ c. cooked)
	100% Whole-Grain Bread (1 slice)

Protein and Dairy	
Beef—round or tenderloin (3 oz.)	Halibut (2–4 oz.)
Cheese—low-fat (1 oz.)	Milk—skim or low-fat (1 c.)
Chicken Breast (2–4 oz.)	Salmon—fresh and wild (2–4 oz.)
Cod (2–4 oz.)	Soy—edamame (½ c. shelled)
Cottage Cheese—low-fat (¼ c.)	Tofu (2–4 oz.)
Egg Whites (3)	Tuna—fresh, wild, or
Greek Yogurt—plain low-fat or	water packed (2–4 oz.)
nonfat (4 oz.)	Turkey Breast—fresh (2–4 oz.)
	Whey Protein (¼ c. or 20 g)

Fats	
Avocado (½ medium)	Oil Cooking Spray—Canola or
Canola Oil (1 tsp.)	Olive (2-second spray)
Flaxseed—milled (2 tbsp.)	Olive Oil—Extra-Virgin (1 tsp.)
Flaxseed Oil (1 tsp.)	Olives (8–10)
Nuts (¼ c.)	Sesame Oil (1 tsp.)

Spices: All spices are approved. Those listed below are some of the most commonly used. Since spices are virtually calorie-free, serving sizes are not an issue.

Basil	Dill	Parsley
Bay leaves	Fennel	Pepper
Cilantro	Lemongrass	Rosemary
Cinnamon	Lemon Zest	Saffron
Cloves	Marjoram	Sage
Coriander	Mint	Tarragon
Cumin	Nutmeg	Thyme
Curry	Oregano	Turmeric

To get the most out of these lists, here are a couple of tips:

1. **Never shop on an empty stomach.** It can cause you to buy more food—and foods that are less healthy—than if you shop on a full stomach.

2. **Stick to the perimeter.** Avoid aisles that contain "junk" or unhealthy foods. Many of these tend to be located in the center aisles of the grocery store. Most whole foods, however, are on the perimeter.

DON'T BE FOOLED

If a food product needs a health claim, such as "heart-healthy," you probably aren't buying a whole food. Remember that some of the healthiest foods you can buy, such as fresh fruit and vegetables, come with no labels, claims, or gimmicks.

---

3. **Balance for energy and sustenance.** For breakfast and morning snacks, incorporate a fruit, a grain, a lean protein, and a healthy fat to create a delicious meal or snack. For lunches, dinners, and afternoon snacks, incorporate a lean protein, a healthy fat, a whole grain, and two or three servings of vegetables in your menu.

4. **Spice up your life.** Use any and all spices in whatever quantity you like: they are savory and calorie free!

THE PERFECT PORTION

It can be difficult to know how much a serving size is without a measuring cup or spoon. To assist you, we have provided a few visual guides, categorized by food type for easy reference.

Fruit and Fibrous Vegetables	
1 c. vegetables, leafy greens, or berries	Baseball Woman's Fist
1 medium-size fruit	Tennis Ball

Grains and Starchy Carbohydrates	
½ c. pasta, rice, cereal	Rounded Handful
1 slice whole grain bread	CD Case
1 potato	Computer Mouse
1 oz. snacks/pretzels	Rounded Handful Tennis Ball
3 c. air-popped popcorn	Three Baseballs

Protein and Dairy	
3 oz. meat or chicken	Deck of Cards Cassette Tape
1 oz. meat or chicken	Matchbook
3 oz. grilled fish	Checkbook
1 oz. hard cheese	Four Dice, Thumb, Tube of Lipstick
1 oz .sliced cheese or deli meat	CD
½ c. nonfat yogurt	Half a Baseball
2 tbsp. hummus	Ping-Pong Ball Shot Glass
½ c. cooked beans	Half a Baseball

Healthy Fats	
1 tbsp. mustard	Thumb
1 tsp. extra-virgin olive oil	Die, Fingertip
¼ c. nuts	Golf Ball, Egg

Source: Lisa R. Young, PhD, RD. *The Portion Teller*, New York: Broadway Books, 2005.

THE PERFECT RECIPE

Cooking and baking can be a challenge when the recipe calls for unhealthy ingredients, such as butter, oil, sugar, etc. To help simplify things, here is a list of key "bad ingredients" and what you can substitute for a healthier version.

Some of these substitutions will create a slightly different consistency or taste, especially when baking. Experiment to find the perfect mixture that works for you. Remember: in most scenarios, there is a healthier, natural substitute for unhealthy and/or processed ingredients.

COOKING

Ingredient	Try
Butter or oil *(½ c.)*	½ c. of 100% natural chicken or vegetable broth, or vinegar
Cornstarch for thickening	Thicken sauce by simmering down to a desired texture
Cream for soup base *(1 c.)*	1 c. skim or 1% milk
	½ c. plain nonfat yogurt
Cream to thicken soup *(1 c.)*	1 c. pureed potatoes or vegetables
Ground beef *(1 lb.)*	1 lb. ground chicken
	1 lb. lean ground turkey (93% or higher)
Mayonnaise (1 tbsp.)	2 tsp. mustard + 1 tsp. olive oil
	1 tbsp. plain nonfat Greek yogurt
Oil-based marinade *(1 tbsp.)*	1 tbsp. citrus juice
	1 tbsp. balsamic vinegar
Salt *(1 tsp.)*	1 tsp. spice
	1 tsp. herb
Sour Cream *(½ c.)*	½ c. plain nonfat Greek yogurt

BAKING

Ingredient	Try
Buttermilk *(1 c.)*	1 c. plain nonfat yogurt
	1 c. skim or 1% milk + 1 tbsp. lemon juice
	1 c. skim or 1% milk + 1 tbsp. white vinegar
Butter or Oil *(1 c.)*	1 c. unsweetened applesauce
Chocolate Chips *(1 c.)*	½ c. mini dark-chocolate chips
	1 c. carob chips
Chocolate *unsweetened (1 oz.)*	3 tbsp. unsweetened cocoa powder + 1 tbsp. vegetable oil
	3 tbsp. of carob powder + 1 tbsp. vegetable oil (reduce sugar by one-quarter)
Corn Syrup *(1 c.)*	⅞ c. honey (baked food will brown more)
Egg *(1 whole)*	2 egg whites
	1 tbsp. ground flaxseed dissolved in 3 tbsp. water
Flour *enriched, white, all-purpose (1 c.)*	⅓ c. 100% whole-grain flour + ⅔ c. unbleached all-purpose flour
Fruit *canned or in light syrup (1 c.)*	1 c. fresh fruit
Ice Cream *(1 c.)*	1 c. frozen yogurt
Milk *whole or 2% (1 c.)*	1 c. 1% or skim milk (respectively)
Nuts *(1 c.)*	½ c. toasted nuts
Sugar *white or brown (1 c.)*	¾ c. honey
	¾ c. maple syrup
	1 c. Sucanat*
Whipped cream *(1 c.)*	3 stiffly beaten egg whites
	¾ c.–1 c. yogurt

CONDIMENTS

Ingredient	Try
Ketchup	fresh salsa
Mayonnaise *(1 tbsp.)*	1 tbsp. roasted garlic
	1 tbsp. plain nonfat yogurt
	1 tbsp. mashed avocado
	1 tbsp. mustard
Sour Cream *(½ c.)*	½ c. plain nonfat Greek yogurt
Soy Sauce *(1 tbsp.)*	1 tbsp. low-sodium soy sauce
Store-bought Salad Dressing	make your own with oils, mustards, vinegars, and honey

* *Sucanat (contraction of "Sugar Cane Natural") is unrefined cane sugar that retains its molasses content. Of all sugars derived from sugar cane, Sucanat ranks highest in nutritional value. Sucanat, however, like all other sugars, is not a significant source of any nutrient other than simple carbohydrates. Sucanat is best used as a substitute for brown sugar.*

8

PREFERRED BRANDS

There will be times when eating whole, all-natural foods isn't possible. You might need to reach for a convenient snack or meal "helper" that provides a quick and easy fix for lunch or dinner. The good news is that the health food market continues to grow, providing more options than ever before. On the following pages, you'll find a list of healthy brands as well as a list of my favorite products within each category. Obviously, this is just a small selection—there are more brands out there! If you prefer to choose brands on your own, here are a few tips:

1. **Long ingredient lists.** If the label has ten or more ingredients, or ingredients you've never heard of, steer clear.

2. **No expiration date.** If a product doesn't have an expiration date, or has an extremely long shelf life, avoid the food. Highly processed baked goods are a perfect example.

3. **When in doubt, choose organics.** Organics are more than just pesticide-free. They usually afford all-around better quality and more natural ingredients.

BREADS, CEREALS, SNACKS
Arrowhead Mills
Barbara's Bakery
Bear Naked
Bob's Red Mill
Campbell Bread Baking Co.
Food Should Taste Good
Gnu Foods
Green's
Health Valley
Hodgson Mill
Kashi Go Lean
Kind Healthy Snacks
Lara Bar
Nature's Path
Odwalla
Sahale Snacks
Somersaults

BOXED, CANNED, JARRED
Amy's Organics
Annie's Naturals
Eden
Green's
Health Valley
Mrs. May's Naturals
Naturade

CONDIMENTS
Amy's Organics
Annie's Naturals
Drew's

DAIRY
Chobani
Fage
Oikos
O'Soy
Stonyfield
Yobaby

DRINKS
GT's Organic & Raw
Honest Beverages
Inko's Tea
Lakewood Organic
Tea's Tea
Yogi

FROZEN FOODS
Amy's Organics
Alexia
Cedarlane
Helen's Kitchen
Kashi

MEATS AND POULTRY
Applewood Farms
Horizon

BRETT'S FAVORITES

Boxed Foods
Annie's Naturals
Organic Macaroni and Cheese

Naturade
Whey Protein—Vanilla

Cereals / Grains
Nature's Path
Flax Plus Multibran Cereal

Bob's Red Mill
Flaxseed Meal

Drinks
Honest Beverages
Honey Green Tea

Yogi
Detox and Bedtime Teas

Fiber Bars
Gnu Foods
Flavor & Fiber Bar
in Espresso Chip

Frozen Foods
Amy's Organics
Margherita Pizza

Cedarlane
Low Fat Beans, Rice, and
Cheese Style Burrito

Snack Bars
Odwalla
Super Protein

Kind Fruit + Nut
Fruit and Nut Delight

Tortilla Chips
Food Should Taste Good
Multigrain Tortilla Chips

Yogurt
Chobani and Oikos
Plain Fat-Free

FINDING PREFERRED BRANDS

Although each region of the country has different retail outlets that carry natural and organic brands, you can find many of the brands listed—plus others—at Whole Foods, Trader Joe's, and local all-natural grocery and food stores. If none are accessible, many brands can be purchased from online retailers, such as ShopOrganic.com, TrueFoodsMarket.com, and Amazon.com.

9

IT'S ALL IN THE LABEL

In chapter 1, *"Keep It Whole, Keep It Natural, Keep It Simple,"* we discussed how to distinguish whole foods from processed foods. We also showed you how to find foods that contain whole grains. To understand the complete picture, however, you also need to know how to read the ingredient list and the nutrition facts label on packaged goods. Doing so will help you to make smart, healthy choices on your own.

HOW TO READ THE INGREDIENT LIST

The ingredient list provides information on what components, spices, and possible chemicals make up the food. Ingredients listed on food labels are presented in weight order. The "heaviest" ingredient is listed first and the "lightest" is listed last. You want to avoid foods that have fat, oils, and sugars (or any derivatives of these ingredients) listed first. Further, if you have never heard of the ingredient or can't pronounce it, there is a good chance it is a chemical or unnatural. As we discussed, whole foods are best; you should be able to recognize all or most of the ingredients listed.

Sometimes sugar, fats, and oils are "disguised" or come in derivatives. The following tables provide a listing of the most common derivatives of these ingredients. Again, if these are listed first on a packaged food, you can be sure they are high in calories, lack nutrition, and are a fattening food.

Sugars	
Bleached Flour*	High-Fructose Corn Syrup
Brown Sugar	Honey
Corn Syrup	Molasses
Dextrose	Sucrose
Fructose	Sugar

Although bleached flour isn't a sugar, it has very little nutritional value, and as a result, the body processes it like a sugar.

Fats and Oils	
Butter	Lard
Coconut Oil	Palm Kernel Oil
Cream	Palm Oil
Hydrogenated and Partially Hydrogenated Oils (Soybean, Vegetable, etc.)	

HOW TO READ THE NUTRITION FACTS LABEL

Nutrition facts labels provide detailed information about foods and products, enabling us to choose the healthiest options. In essence, they deliver the wherewithal for us to understand how different products stack up against one another. Please refer to the nutrition facts label shown on the next page. Reference numbers are provided for each section, together with accompanying descriptions/explanations.

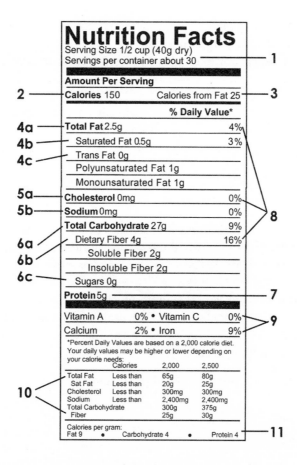

1. **Serving Size.** The *serving size* delineates the recommended portion per serving. Here are some tips.

   - **When in Doubt, Measure.** If you aren't used to measuring or weighing your food, do so until you become comfortable with standard portion sizes.
   - **Nutritional Values and Number of Servings.** If you eat more or less than the recommended serving size, the rest of the label information needs to be adjusted accordingly;

e.g., if you have two times the serving, all nutritional values must be multiplied by two.

- **Compare Apples with Apples.** When comparing foods, be sure your comparison is based on equal portion sizes.

2. **Calories.** *Calories* provide you with an "energy measure" to be derived from each serving. Remember: the number of servings consumed determines the number of calories ingested. For instance, if you have two portions of a food, double the calories listed. Here is a good gauge to judge if something is high or low in calories:

- **Low-Calorie Food** = 40 calories per serving
- **Moderate-Calorie Food** = 100 calories per serving
- **High-Calorie Food** = 400 calories or more per serving

3. **Calories from Fat.** This indicates the number of fat calories per recommended serving. Each gram of fat is worth approximately 9 calories. You can calculate this on your own by using the following equation:

Calculation 1: Number of Calories from Fat

$$\text{9 calories per gram of fat} \quad \times \quad \text{number of grams of fat} \quad = \quad \text{approximate number of calories from fat}$$

In our example, the product contains 2.5 grams of fat. To get the number of calories from fat, we use Calculation 1:

$$\text{9 calories per gram of fat} \quad \times \quad \text{2.5 grams of fat} \quad = \quad \text{approximately } \textbf{23 calories* are from fat}$$

Remember, this is an approximation. The package information may not exactly match your own calculation.

In chapter 4, *"Enjoy Healthy Fats,"* we mentioned that 20 to 30 percent of calories should come from fat. To calculate this figure, use the following equation:

Calculation 2: Percent of Calories from Fat

$$\frac{\text{number of calories from fat}}{\text{total number of calories}} = \text{percent of calories from fat}$$

Using the number of calories we derived in Calculation 1, we calculate the percentage of calories from fat:

$$\frac{23 \text{ calories from fat}}{150 \text{ total calories}} = \textbf{15.3 percent} \text{ of calories from fat}$$

As you can see, our example is a low-fat food. A good rule of thumb for daily fat caloric intake is a maximum of 30 fat calories per 100 calories of food.

4. **Total Fat Breakdown.** This section indicates how healthy or unhealthy the fats are in a product.

   4a. **Total Fat.** *Total fat* explains how much of both good (monounsaturated and polyunsaturated) and bad fats (saturated and trans) are in the food. As mentioned previously, you should have no more than 3 grams of fat per 100 calories.

   4b. **Saturated Fat.** A "bad fat," *saturated fat* is found in foods such as butter, margarine, fats from meat and pork, full-fat dairy products, eggs, palm and coconut oils, and many fast foods. It is best to avoid or strictly limit foods that have saturated fat. Daily intake should be no more than 10 percent of daily caloric intake (less than 1 gram per 100 calories). In our example, it is evident that this product is low in saturated fat.

4c. **Trans Fat.** Also a "bad fat," *trans fat* is created during cooking and/or processing. These fats are often found in commercially baked products and should be eliminated from your diet. In our example, the product contains no trans fat.

In analyzing this product's fat content, "healthy fat" predominates, with 1 gram of fat coming from monounsaturated and 1 gram coming from polyunsaturated fats.

Note: Although our sample nutrition facts label shows both polyunsaturated fat and monounsaturated fat content, some nutrition facts labels do not provide this information. In these cases, the best way to determine if the product contains unhealthy fats is to compare the *saturated fat* content with the *total fat* content. If the numbers are equal (or close to one another), you can be relatively certain that there are very little, if any, healthy fats in the product. Consequently, it is best to avoid the food.

5. **Cholesterol and Sodium.** When comparing packaged foods, make sure that they represent comparable serving sizes. Then look at the cholesterol and sodium. Always opt for the food that has the least amount of both cholesterol and sodium per serving.

   5a. **Cholesterol.** The *cholesterol* number provides you with the amount of dietary cholesterol in each serving. Dietary cholesterol raises levels of LDL, which contributes to heart disease. To be safe, it is best to eat no more than 300 mg of cholesterol per day.

   5b. **Sodium.** The *sodium* number provides the amount of sodium in a serving. It is best to eat no more than 2,400 mg per day.

6. **Carbohydrate Breakdown.** This section indicates the quality of carbohydrate in a product.

6a. **Total Carbohydrate.** This section includes simple carbs and sugars, as well as complex carbs and fiber. Each gram of carbohydrate is worth approximately four calories. To evaluate the number of calories that come from carbohydrates, the calculation follows:

Calculation 3: Number of Calories from Carbohydrates

$$\text{4 calories per gram of carb} \quad \times \quad \begin{matrix} \text{number of} \\ \text{grams} \\ \text{of carbs} \end{matrix} \quad = \quad \begin{matrix} \text{approximate} \\ \text{number of calories} \\ \text{from carbs} \end{matrix}$$

In this case, the label shows that the product contains 27 grams of carbohydrates. To get the number of calories, we use Calculation 3:

$$\text{4 calories} \quad \times \quad \begin{matrix} \text{27 grams} \\ \text{of carbs} \end{matrix} \quad = \quad \begin{matrix} \text{approximately} \\ \textbf{108 calories} \\ \text{from carbs} \end{matrix}$$

Ideally, 40 to 60 percent of calories should come from carbohydrates. To calculate the percentage of calories specific to carbohydrates in this product, use the following equation:

Calculation 4: Percent of Calories from Carbohydrates

$$\frac{\text{number of calories from carbs}}{\text{total number of calories}} \quad = \quad \begin{matrix} \text{percent of calories} \\ \text{from carbs} \end{matrix}$$

Again, in this case, using the number of calories derived from Calculation 3, the percentage of calories from carbohydrates is calculated as follows:

$$\frac{\text{108 calories from carbs}}{\text{150 total calories}} \quad = \quad \begin{matrix} \textbf{72 percent} \text{ of} \\ \text{calories from carbs} \end{matrix}$$

6b. **Dietary Fiber.** The *dietary fiber* tells you how much fiber is in a serving of the packaged food. Found in carbohydrates such as whole grains, fruits, vegetables, and beans, fiber is an important nutrient. Often, the label will provide quantities of both insoluble and soluble fiber. A few things to remember:

- Try to eat 25 to 35 grams of fiber per day.
- Aim for an average of 2 grams of fiber per 100 calories.
- The higher the fiber content, the lower the sugar content.

6c. **Sugars.** Carbohydrates also contain simple sugars. When looking at nutrition facts labels, this number should be low in relationship to the number of total carbohydrates. The closer the number of grams of sugar is to the total number of grams of carbohydrate, the less fiber, the more empty calories, and the less filling is the food. It is best to consume no more than 32 to 36 grams of added sugar a day. ("Added sugar" doesn't include sugar naturally found in whole fruit or dairy products.)

As you can see, our example is a high-carbohydrate food, but it is high in fiber and low in sugars. As a result, it contains little to no empty calories and is quite filling because of its high fiber content.

In calculating daily caloric intake, eat between 10 grams and 15 grams of carbohydrates per 100 calories of food.

7. **Protein.** *Protein* indicates the total grams of protein in a serving. It is always advisable to maintain a balance of protein, carbohydrates, and fats in a meal or snack. If the product considered doesn't contain protein, try to combine it with another food that does. Each gram of protein is worth approximately four calories. To calculate the number of calories of protein in a food, use the following equation:

Calculation 5: Number of Calories from Protein

		number of grams of protein	=	approximate number of calories from protein
4 calories	x			

In our example, the product contains 5 grams of protein. Calculate the number of calories from protein, as follows:

		5 grams of protein	=	approximately **20 calories** from protein
4 calories	x			

In chapter 3, *"Pack Lean Proteins into Every Meal,"* we stated that 20 to 40 percent of your calories should come from protein. To calculate the percentage of protein calories in this product, use the following:

Calculation 6: Percent of Calories from Protein

$$\frac{\text{number of calories from protein}}{\text{total number of calories}} = \text{percent of calories from protein}$$

Using the number of calories derived in Calculation 5, the percentage of calories from protein is calculated as follows:

$$\frac{20 \text{ calories from protein}}{150 \text{ total calories}} = \textbf{13 percent} \text{ of calories from protein}$$

As is evident, this example is a low-protein food. For daily caloric intake, a good rule of thumb: eat 5 to 10 grams of protein per 100 calories of food.

8. **Percent Daily Values.** The *daily values* listing shows how much of your recommended daily allowance of fat,

cholesterol, sodium, carbohydrates, and fiber is provided in a single serving. Note, however, that percentages are based on a 2,000-calorie diet. Generally, a value of 5 percent is considered low; a value of 20 percent high. If you consume more or less than 2,000 calories a day, these percentages may change; therefore, use these numbers solely as a guide.

9. **Vitamins and Minerals.** These numbers tell what percentage of the recommended daily intake of vitamins and minerals are in a serving of the product. During the course of the day, you should aim to reach 100 percent of all required vitamins and minerals. To ensure you reach this goal, it is recommended that you take a multivitamin.

10. **Recommended Amounts.** This provides a total recommended daily amount of each nutrient for both a 2,000-calorie diet and a 2,500-calorie diet. If you need to consume more or less than 2,000 or 2,500 calories a day to maintain a healthy body weight, the recommended amounts for fat, cholesterol, sodium, and carbohydrates will change.

11. **Calories per Gram.** As we have explained, fat, carbohydrates, and protein all have different caloric values per gram. This part of the label reminds you of the caloric weight of each. It is best to choose foods that are well balanced and that contain all nutrients.

NUTRITION REQUIREMENTS SUMMARY

To simplify some of the details presented in this chapter, the following chart provides you with a summary of the caloric weight of each nutrient (when applicable), the number of grams you should incorporate into your diet, and the overall percentage of calories that should be dedicated to the nutrient (when applicable). The number of grams you should eat and the percentage of daily caloric intake represent the same concept in two different ways. Use whichever is easiest for you to remember, understand, and follow.

Nutrient	Calories per gram*	Number of grams you should consume	Percent of daily caloric intake
Fat	9	2.5–3.25 grams *per 100 calories*	20–30%
Saturated Fat	-	< 1 gram *per 100 calories*	< 10%
Cholesterol	-	< 300mg *per day*	-
Sodium	-	< 2,400mg *per day*	-
Carbohydrates	4	10–15 grams *per 100 calories*	40–60%
Fiber	-	25–35 grams *per day*	
Sugar (added)	-	32–36 grams *per day*	
Protein	4	5–10 grams *per 100 calories*	20–40%

* This is an approximate number, but is a standard in the industry.

10

RECIPES

The following recipes were created to be well balanced and adhere to most, if not all, of the "GET REAL" principles. They include tasty foods to satisfy your appetite and provide the essential nutrients your body requires. Cooking from scratch is a much healthier option than buying premade alternatives because the manufacturing process introduces chemicals, preservatives, and additives that negatively impact our bodies.

To get the most out of this section, use these recipes as a guide and modify them to suit your taste. If, for instance, you prefer salmon instead of chicken, you can substitute it in any of the recipes. Just remember: use alternatives that have similar nutritional values (refer to chapter 7, *"Practice Makes Perfect,"* for appropriate substitutions)!

With the exception of fibrous vegetables, ALWAYS SUBSTITUTE, never add. For instance, if you prefer avocado to cheese, REPLACE the cheese in a recipe; do not simply add the avocado to it. Adding ingredients will throw off the nutritional balance. Again, refer to chapter 7, *"Practice Makes Perfect,"* for a clear understanding of which foods can be substituted safely and appropriately.

Each recipe provides nutritional information per serving to clearly illustrate why the recipe is especially healthy and how the ingredients combine to create well-balanced, nutritious, and filling meals. The ingredients in any single-serving recipe can be doubled, tripled, etc., to create more servings.

BREAKFAST

Breakfast is the most important meal of your day! Each of the following recipes is well balanced to help you get a healthy start. Each meal is between 250 and 375 calories and is high in fiber and protein to keep you feeling satisfied throughout the morning.

APPLE-BANANA PROTEIN SHAKE

Protein shakes are an easy and tasty breakfast. You can mix whey protein powder with fruit, vegetables, milk, or water to concoct a mixture you enjoy. This is one of my personal favorites.

Ingredients
1 apple—peeled and cored
½ banana
¼ cup vanilla whey protein (unsweetened—Naturade)
1-½ teaspoons cinnamon
¼ cup old-fashioned rolled oats
1 cup water

Directions: Blend until smooth. Enjoy!

Makes 1 Serving

NUTRITION PER SERVING Calories = 306							
	Total Fat	Sat. Fat	Poly. Fat	Mono. Fat	Carbs	Fiber	Sugars	Protein
grams	2.8 g	0.9 g	0.6 g	0.4 g	55 g	8.6 g	25 g	20 g
% of calories	8%				66%			26%

MIXED BERRY PROTEIN SHAKE

Berries are high in antioxidants and other vitamins and minerals. If fresh berries are out of season, use frozen. Look at the ingredient list, however, to be sure there are no additives or other ingredients besides the berries!

Ingredients
¼ cup raspberries
¼ cup blackberries
¼ cup blueberries
¼ cup strawberries
2 tablespoons ground flaxseed
¼ cup vanilla whey protein
   (unsweetened—Naturade)
1 cup skim milk

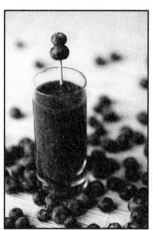

Directions: Blend until smooth.

Makes 1 Serving

	Total Fat	Sat. Fat	Poly. Fat	Mono. Fat	Carbs	Fiber	Sugars	Protein
NUTRITION PER SERVING Calories = 288								
grams	6.2 g	0.7 g	5.0 g	0.3 g	30 g	8.5 g	22 g	30.4 g
% of calories	20%				40%			40%

GRILLED BREAKFAST SANDWICH

With more fiber and less fat, this is a much healthier version of the traditional egg sandwich. Flavorwise, however, it is as tasty as ever!

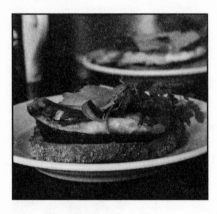

Ingredients
Canola oil spray
¼ cup yellow onion—
   chopped
¼ cup green pepper—
   chopped
2 egg whites
Salt and pepper to taste
2 slices 100% whole-grain
   bread
2 slices lean Canadian
   bacon
1 slice low-fat cheddar or
   Colby cheese

Directions: Spray nonstick pan with 1-second spray of canola oil and heat on medium. Cook onions and peppers until tender. Remove from pan and set aside. Spray pan again with 1-second spray of canola oil. Cook eggs for a minute. Add mixture of onions and peppers. Add salt and pepper to taste. Stir until eggs are cooked through.

Toast bread. Set eggs aside and cook Canadian bacon for about a minute on each side. Layer ingredients on 1 piece of toast in following order: 1 slice Canadian bacon, eggs, second piece of Canadian bacon, and cheese. Press other piece of toast on top. Spray pan 1 more time with 1-second spray of canola oil. Cook sandwich on each side for 15 seconds. Remove from pan and eat immediately.

Makes 1 Serving

NUTRITION PER SERVING Calories = 369								
	Total Fat	Sat. Fat	Poly. Fat	Mono. Fat	Carbs	Fiber	Sugars	Protein
grams	13 g	3.7 g	1.9 g	6.2 g	30 g	5.2 g	7 g	33 g
% of calories	31%				32%			37%

HARVEST OATMEAL

As a breakfast choice, it is hard to dispute oatmeal's popularity. Oats provide many benefits, including fiber and the power to lower cholesterol. Using 100% apple juice to sweeten the taste and walnuts to provide some healthy fat and protein, this is a healthier option than instant or traditionally "doctored" versions.

Ingredients
½ cup water
¼ cup 100% apple juice
¼ cup old-fashioned rolled oats
2 tablespoons raisins or dried cranberries
2 tablespoons chopped walnuts
½ teaspoon cinnamon
Pinch nutmeg

Directions: In a small pot, bring water and apple juice to a boil. Stir in oats, raisins (or dried cranberries), chopped walnuts, cinnamon, and nutmeg. Cook mixture for about 5 minutes over medium heat, or until it has thickened to a good consistency. Stir before serving.

Makes 1 Serving

	Total Fat	Sat. Fat	Poly. Fat	Mono. Fat	Carbs	Fiber	Sugars	Protein
NUTRITION PER SERVING Calories = 266								
grams	10.4 g	0.9 g	2.8 g	6.0 g	39.7 g	5.3 g	6 g	7.6 g
% of calories	33%				57%			10%

MUSHROOM AND ASPARAGUS EGG-WHITE OMELET

Made with egg whites, this omelet is low in fat and cholesterol. Pair with multigrain toast to make this a well-balanced breakfast.

Ingredients
Canola oil cooking spray
¼ cup fresh mushrooms
3 fresh asparagus spears—chopped
3 egg whites
1 ounce fat-free feta cheese (1 cubic inch)
Salt and pepper to taste
2 slices 100% multigrain bread
½ tablespoon raspberry preserves

Directions: Spray a skillet with 1-second spray of canola oil cooking spray. Cook mushrooms and asparagus so that mushrooms are slightly tender and asparagus is bright green. Remove from heat and set aside.

Spray skillet once more with a 1-second spray of canola oil. Add egg whites. Cook until eggs are firm on bottom (top should still look wet, but not move). Use a spatula to flip over eggs to cook other side.

Crumble fat-free feta evenly on top of one half of the eggs. Spread cooked mushrooms and asparagus on top of feta and eggs. Add salt and pepper to taste. Fold eggs over to create a half-moon omelet and cook for 1 minute. Meanwhile, toast bread. Flip omelet over onto other side and let sit for another minute. Spread preserves onto toast and serve immediately.

Makes 1 Serving

	Total Fat	Sat. Fat	Poly. Fat	Mono. Fat	Carbs	Fiber	Sugars	Protein
NUTRITION PER SERVING **Calories = 275**								
grams	7 g	1.1 g	1.5 g	3.7 g	27 g	5 g	5 g	26 g
% of calories	22%				40%			38%

PLEASANTLY SURPRISING WHOLE-GRAIN PANCAKES

Normally, I don't like pancakes. These, however, surprised me with their hearty and delicious flavor. Full of whole grains, protein, calcium, and an array of vitamins, these pancakes will give you a sweet start to a wonderful day.

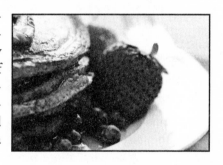

Ingredients

1 cup whole-wheat flour
½ cup old-fashioned rolled oats
¼ cup whole-grain cornmeal
3 tablespoons flaxseed meal
1 teaspoon baking powder
½ teaspoon baking soda

1 teaspoon cinnamon
½ teaspoon nutmeg
3 tablespoons pure maple syrup
1 whole egg—beaten
1½ cups low-fat buttermilk
4 cups fresh berries of your choice

Directions: In large bowl, mix flour, oats, and grain meals with baking powder, baking soda, cinnamon, and nutmeg. Make a well in center and pour in maple syrup, egg, and buttermilk. Mix until dry ingredients are moist.

Heat large, nonstick skillet at medium heat. Once heated through, drop spoonfuls of batter onto skillet and cook until edges are dry. Flip pancakes and cook until other side is slightly browned. Serve with fresh berries.

Makes 4 Servings

NUTRITION PER SERVING								
Calories = 340								
	Total Fat	Sat. Fat	Poly. Fat	Mono. Fat	Carbs	Fiber	Sugars	Protein
Grams	6.3 g	1.4 g	2.6 g	1.5 g	63.1 g	11.7 g	19.6 g	13 g
% of calories	16%				70%			14%

GREEK YOGURT PARFAIT

Traditional yogurt parfaits are loaded with carbohydrates and sugar. They also lack protein and rely on refined sugars for sweetness. This version has more protein and less sugar, and with ground flaxseed, it provides a healthy dose of omega-3s.

Ingredients
1 cup mixed berries (use frozen if fresh are out of season)
1 cup plain nonfat Greek yogurt
2 tablespoons ground flaxseed
¼ cup old-fashioned rolled oats

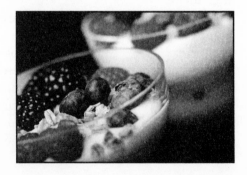

Directions: Mix berries, yogurt, ground flaxseed, and oats.

Makes 1 Serving

	Total Fat	Sat. Fat	Poly. Fat	Mono. Fat	Carbs	Fiber	Sugars	Protein
NUTRITION PER SERVING Calories = 321								
grams	6 g	0 g	5.0 g	1.5 g	43 g	11 g	19 g	30 g
% of calories	17%				46%			37%

LUNCH AND DINNER

The recipes in this section can be used interchangeably between lunch and dinner. To save time, make big batches and store them for the week. Each meal is between 250 and 400 calories.

SIMPLE BAKED CHICKEN (SBC)

To make lunch and dinner especially healthy, quick, and easy, I recommend eating large salads with about 2 to 4 ounces of protein. Bake a batch of chicken on a Sunday night to include in lunches or dinners throughout the week. Pre-planning meals this way helps with shopping and portion control.

Either of the Simple Baked Chicken recipes can be paired with any salad or meal that calls for chicken.

Ingredients
Canola oil cooking spray
1 pound skinless, boneless chicken breasts—2 to 3 breasts
1 cup chicken broth

Spices for SBC—Italian Style	Spices for SBC—Indian Style
2 tablespoons paprika	2 tablespoons curry powder
2 tablespoons dried oregano	1 tablespoon cumin
Salt and pepper to taste	1 tablespoon turmeric
2 tablespoons fresh parsley	1 tablespoon caraway seeds
	1 teaspoon paprika

Directions: Preheat oven to 350°F. Spray bottom of baking dish with canola oil. Place chicken in a single layer and pour chicken broth over it. Depending on the style you choose, layer spices on each breast in the order listed—e.g., for Italian, paprika, oregano, salt and pepper to taste, and, finally, parsley. Cover and bake for 15 minutes, and then uncover and bake for another 15 minutes, or until done. When done, cut chicken into meal-sized portions. Refrigerate leftovers immediately.

Makes 5 Servings

NUTRITION PER SERVING Calories = 139								
	Total Fat	Sat. Fat	Poly. Fat	Mono. Fat	Carbs	Fiber	Sugars	Protein
grams	3.1 g	0.9 g	0.7 g	1.2 g	0 g	0 g	0 g	25.8 g
% of calories	20%				0%			80%

PEASANT SALAD WITH CHICKEN

This salad is a take on the traditional Greek salad. Without the use of lettuce as a filler, however, it is heartier, tastier, and more nutritious than traditional Greek salads.

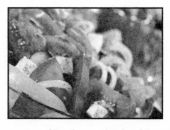

Ingredients

1 cup grape tomatoes—cut in half

¾ cup cucumber—sliced and quartered

½ cup red onion—chopped medium

½ cup red pepper—chopped

½ cup green pepper—chopped

¼ cup fat-free feta cheese—crumbled

2 ounces diced, cooked, skinless chicken breast (see "Italian Style SBC")

1 teaspoon extra-virgin olive oil

1 teaspoon lemon juice

2 tablespoons red wine vinegar

1 tablespoon fresh basil—chopped

Salt, pepper, fresh parsley, and dried oregano to taste

Directions: Put tomatoes, cucumber, red onion, red pepper, green pepper, feta, and chicken breast in a bowl. Next, drizzle olive oil, lemon juice, and vinegar over mixture. Add basil, salt, pepper, parsley, and oregano to taste, and mix. Eat immediately.

Makes 1 Serving

	Total Fat	Sat. Fat	Poly. Fat	Mono. Fat	Carbs	Fiber	Sugars	Protein
NUTRITION PER SERVING Calories = 327								
grams	6.3 g	1.1 g	1.0 g	3.6 g	26 g	6.1 g	12 g	41 g
% of calories	17%				33%			50%

TABOULE SALAD WITH SALMON

If you can't find cracked bulgur, you can buy Near East packaged taboule, which provides you with the "seasoning mix" and cracked wheat in one package. Fresh taboule, however, is preferable.

Ingredients

½ cup boiling water
½ cup cracked bulgur
6 ounces wild salmon*
2 tablespoons lemon
    juice
½ cup fresh parsley
Pepper to taste

1 tomato—coarsely chopped
3 scallions—finely chopped
1 teaspoon fresh minced garlic
1 tablespoon extra-virgin
    olive oil
Salt to taste
1 teaspoon dry oregano

Directions: Preheat oven to 350°F. In medium bowl, stir boiling water into cracked bulgur. Cover and refrigerate for 30 minutes. Put salmon in glass baking dish with a cover. Pour 1 tablespoon of lemon juice over salmon and sprinkle with ¼ cup fresh parsley and ground pepper. Cover and bake at 350°F for 10 minutes per inch of thickness.

Combine tomatoes, scallions, garlic, ¼ cup parsley, 1 table-spoon lemon juice, and olive oil with bulgur from refrigerator. Season mixture to taste with salt, pepper, and oregano. Mix well. When salmon is finished, remove and serve with taboule. Taboule can be served chilled or at room temperature.

Makes 2 Servings

	Total Fat	Sat. Fat	Poly. Fat	Mono. Fat	Carbs	Fiber	Sugars	Protein
NUTRITION PER SERVING Calories = 321								
grams	11 g	1.6 g	2.4 g	6 g	30.6 g	7.7 g	3 g	26.5 g
% of calories	31%				36%			34%

* NOTE: Salmon should be baked in a covered dish at 350°F for 10 minutes per inch (thickness) of fish.

PROTEIN POWER PEANUT BUTTER RICE

I admit that I don't like tofu. I have very little interest in it. The tofu in this recipe, however, is meant to be so subtle in flavor that you won't even know it is part of the dish. If you are absolutely resistant to tofu as an ingredient, you can substitute 1 tablespoon coconut milk plus 10 ounces of nonfat Greek yogurt for the tofu.

Ingredients
1 cup brown rice
3 cups broccoli flowerets—cut into bite-size pieces
2 cups green beans
½ cup lima beans
2 teaspoons sesame seed oil
2 tablespoons soy sauce
1 package silken tofu (16 ounces)
2 tablespoons all-natural peanut butter—smooth (no sugar added)

Directions: Combine rice with 2 cups of water in a small pot with a tight-fitting lid. Bring to a boil. Stir and cover. Reduce heat to simmer and cook for 50 minutes.

After 30 minutes, over low heat, stir-fry the broccoli, green beans, and lima beans in the sesame oil and soy sauce until soft (about 20 minutes). Just before broccoli is done, blend together tofu and peanut butter until creamy. Then add to the broccoli. Serve over rice.

Makes 6 Servings

	Total Fat	Sat. Fat	Poly. Fat	Mono. Fat	Carbs	Fiber	Sugars	Protein
NUTRITION PER SERVING Calories = 279								
grams	8 g	1.4 g	3.4 g	2.8 g	40 g	6 g	3 g	14 g
% of calories	25%				58%			17%

TUNA BOATS AND BUOYS

Although canned tuna is not as nutritious as fresh tuna, it is still a healthy option as compared to other canned foods. This is a great summer lunch that is refreshing and filling—as well as a fabulous light Sunday supper.

Ingredients

2 beefsteak tomatoes
Salt and pepper
1 can solid white tuna—7 ounces
    (packed in spring water)
¼ cup yellow onion—minced
2 celery stalks—chopped fine
1 tablespoon lemon juice
1 tablespoon Dijon mustard
2 teaspoons extra-virgin olive oil
1 tablespoon capers
2 slices 100%
    whole-grain bread
1 cucumber—peeled, seeded,
    and cut in half lengthwise

Directions: Cut off tops of tomatoes and remove cores and seeds. Sprinkle salt inside each and place upside down on a paper towel.

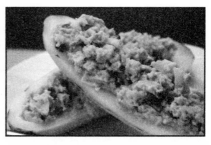

Drain tuna and pulse in food processor to a fine consistency. Place onion, celery, tuna, lemon juice, Dijon mustard, olive oil, and capers in a medium bowl and mix well. Add salt and pepper to taste.

Toast bread. Fill tuna salad into tomatoes and cucumber halves. Serve immediately.

Makes 2 Servings

	Total Fat	Sat. Fat	Poly. Fat	Mono. Fat	Carbs	Fiber	Sugars	Protein
NUTRITION PER SERVING Calories = 260								
grams	7.1 g	1.1 g	1.5 g	3.9 g	22.4 g	5.4 g	8 g	41 g
% of calories	24%				33%			43%

EASY, FILLING VEGGIE SOUP

Make this ahead of time and keep it in the fridge to heat up for a quick, delicious lunch or dinner. With tons of vegetables, it provides vitamins and minerals, and the beans and barley contain protein and fiber to keep you full.

Ingredients

4 cups chicken or vegetable broth

2 medium tomatoes—coarsely chopped

1 yellow onion—coarsely chopped

2 cloves garlic—minced

2 stalks celery—finely chopped
2 carrots—peeled and
  thinly sliced
¼ teaspoon chili powder
1 teaspoon fresh dill
1 teaspoon dried thyme
1 teaspoon salt
1 cup hulled barley (soaked
  overnight)

1 can kidney beans (15 ounces)
  —drained and rinsed
1 cup corn kernels (cut off the
  ear or frozen)
2 cups zucchini—sliced
2 tablespoons fresh parsley—
  chopped

Directions: Put chicken broth, tomatoes, onion, garlic, celery, carrots, chili powder, dill, thyme, salt, and presoaked barley into a large pot. Bring to a boil. Cover and reduce to medium heat. Let simmer for 30 minutes. Add in beans, corn, zucchini, and parsley, and simmer for another 10 minutes, so as to leave the zucchini a bit crunchy.

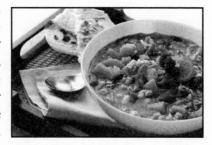

Makes 4 Servings

NUTRITION PER SERVING								
Calories = 354								
	Total Fat	Sat. Fat	Poly. Fat	Mono. Fat	Carbs	Fiber	Sugars	Protein
grams	3.1 g	0.7 g	1.3 g	1.0 g	72.3 g	18.6 g	10.5 g	15.4 g
% of calories	8%				77%			15%

SPINACH, RAISIN, AND CHICKPEA SALAD WITH CHICKEN

Ingredients
3 cups baby spinach
2 tablespoons raisins
$^1/_3$ cup cucumber—chopped
¼ cup red onion—chopped
$^1/_3$ cup canned chickpeas—drained and rinsed
3 ounces skinless chicken breast—diced (see SBC)
½ tablespoon extra-virgin olive oil
1 tablespoon balsamic vinegar
Salt and pepper to taste

Directions: Place spinach, raisins, cucumber, red onion, drained chickpeas, and cubed chicken in a bowl. Next, drizzle olive oil and balsamic vinegar over mixture. Salt and pepper to taste. Mix well.

Makes 1 Serving

	Total Fat	Sat. Fat	Poly. Fat	Mono. Fat	Carbs	Fiber	Sugars	Protein
NUTRITION PER SERVING Calories = 345								
grams	9.2 g	1.4 g	1.5 g	5.4 g	41.2 g	7.1 g	13.7 g	27 g
% of calories	24%				45%			31%

SPINACH AND ARUGULA WITH PAN-SEARED TUNA

Ingredients

3 ounces tuna steak
Salt and pepper
2 cups baby spinach
2 cups arugula
¼ cup red onion—thinly
  sliced
½ cup chickpeas—
  drained and rinsed
¼ cup cucumber—diced
Canola oil cooking spray

Ingredients—Dressing*

1 tablespoon fresh ground
  ginger root
3 tablespoons rice vinegar
¼ cup sesame oil
1½ garlic cloves—minced
¼ cup low-sodium soy sauce
2 tablespoons water
1 tablespoon honey

Directions: Preheat broiler. Spray tuna on each side with 1-second spray of canola oil, and season both sides with salt and pepper to taste. Put tuna into broiling pan.

Mix spinach, arugula, red onion, chickpeas, and cucumber in a bowl and set aside.

Dressing. (You can prepare ahead and store in refrigerator.) Thoroughly mix ginger, rice vinegar, sesame oil, garlic, soy sauce, water, and honey, until honey is well dissolved. Set aside.

Broil tuna steaks. Medium rare is about 2–3 minutes on each side. When done, slice tuna into ⅛-inch slices. Add sliced tuna into salad bowl. Add about 1 to 1½ tablespoons of the dressing. Toss well. Eat immediately.

Makes 1 Serving

* *The dressing recipe makes about 10 servings. A single serving = approximately 1 to 1½ tablespoons of the mixture.*

	Total Fat	Sat. Fat	Poly. Fat	Mono. Fat	Carbs	Fiber	Sugars	Protein
NUTRITION PER SERVING Calories = 337								
grams	8 g	1.2 g	3.4 g	2.6 g	37.7 g	8.1 g	5 g	29 g
% of calories	21%				45%			34%

REAL FRUIT-VEGETABLE SALAD

With the fresh fruit and vegetables in this salad, you will get a whole host of wonderful vitamins, minerals, and antioxidants. The almonds and beans provide healthy fat and protein to balance out the carbs.

Ingredients—Dressing
1 tablespoon chopped green onions
¾ cup raspberries (fresh is best, frozen works)
¼ cup water
¼ cup raspberry vinegar
1 tablespoon Dijon mustard
$^1/_8$ teaspoon sea salt
2 drops stevia—optional

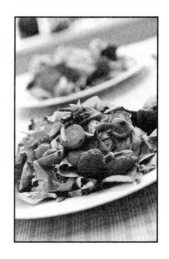

Ingredients—Salad
16 ounces spinach leaves
1 cup snap peas
1 cup alfalfa sprouts
½ cup black beans
1 tomato—chopped
½ orange—peeled and sliced
¼ cup almonds—chopped
Pepper to taste

Directions: Blend the dressing ingredients together. In a bowl, combine the salad ingredients. Then pour the dressing over the salad and toss. Serve immediately.

Makes 2 Servings

NUTRITION PER SERVING Calories = 303							
	Total Fat	Sat. Fat	Poly. Fat	Mono. Fat	Carbs	Fiber	Sugars	Protein
grams	11 g	1 g	3.1 g	6.1 g	39 g	17.5 g	11 g	18 g
% of calories	31%				51%			18%

AVOCADO AND TOMATO SALAD WITH CHICKEN

Although high in fat, the avocados in this salad provide a healthy dose of monounsaturated fat.

Ingredients
½ cup diced avocado (about ¹/₃ of an avocado)
2 large tomatoes—chopped coarsely
½ cup chopped red onion
3 ounces skinless chicken breast—diced (see SBC recipe)
1 teaspoon extra-virgin olive oil
Juice of ½ lime
Salt, pepper, and parsley

Directions: In bowl, put diced avocado, chopped tomatoes, chopped onions, and cubed chicken. Next, drizzle olive oil and lime juice over mixture. Add salt, pepper, and parsley to taste; mix well.

Makes 1 Serving

NUTRITION PER SERVING Calories = 305								
	Total Fat	Sat. Fat	Poly. Fat	Mono. Fat	Carbs	Fiber	Sugars	Protein
grams	13 g	2.0 g	1.8 g	8.1 g	26 g	8.8 g	13 g	24 g
% of calories	37%				31%			32%

MEDITERRANEAN PENNE

This vegetarian dish provides a complete protein. You can replace the beans with a 3-ounce skinless, boneless chicken breast or piece of salmon if you would like a higher dose of protein and fewer carbs.

Ingredients
½ cup whole-wheat penne pasta—dry
½ tablespoon extra-virgin olive oil
1 tablespoon balsamic vinegar
1 clove garlic—minced
½ cup asparagus—chopped
½ cup cherry tomatoes—halved
Dried oregano
¼ cup white cannellini beans—
    drained and rinsed
¼ cup fresh chopped basil
Salt and pepper
1 tablespoon grated parmesan

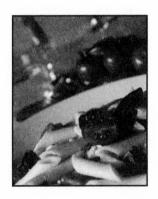

Directions: Bring 1 quart of water to a boil. Add penne and cook for 9 to 10 minutes or until done. Drain the water but do NOT rinse pasta.

In the same pot, add olive oil, balsamic vinegar, garlic, chopped asparagus, tomatoes, oregano, and beans. Stir. Add basil, salt, and pepper to taste. Serve with a sprinkle of parmesan.

Makes 1 Serving

NUTRITION PER SERVING Calories = 397							
	Total Fat	Sat. Fat	Poly. Fat	Mono. Fat	Carbs	Fiber	Sugars	Protein
grams	10.1 g	1.9 g	0.9 g	5.4 g	63.4 g	11.4 g	7.8 g	16 g
% of calories	23%				62%			15%

FARM-FRESH ITALIAN CALZONES

Traditional calzones may conjure up images of unhealthy, greasy food, but this version will change your perception. Not only are these healthy, but they are as tasty and delicious as their greasier alternatives. Experiment with different fillings to get a variety of flavors

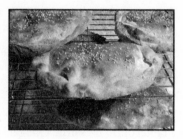

Ingredients—Pizza Dough

1 package active dry yeast (7 g)
1 cup warm water (100–110°F)
2 cups whole-wheat flour

¼ cup wheat germ
1 teaspoon salt
1 tablespoon honey

Ingredients—Sauce

2 large ripe tomatoes—diced
¾ medium onion—diced
¼ cup fresh chopped basil
1 teaspoon dried tarragon

½ teaspoon salt
1 teaspoon red pepper flakes
1 teaspoon dried oregano
1 clove garlic—minced

Ingredients—Filling

¾ medium onion—thinly sliced
1½ bell peppers—julienned (red and orange work best)
¾ pound chicken breasts
Parchment paper
2 egg whites—beaten

Directions: Preheat the oven to 350°F.

Pizza Dough. Dissolve yeast in 1 cup warm water. Let stand for 5 minutes. Spoon out whole-wheat flour into a large mixing bowl. Add wheat germ, salt, honey, and yeast mixture. Mix with the bread hook of an electric mixer for 3 minutes on low. Let sit for 2 minutes; then mix again on low for 3 more minutes. Let it sit as you prepare the sauce.

Sauce. Place the diced tomatoes and onions in a small saucepan on low heat. Add spices, crushing them between your palms as you sprinkle them into the tomatoes. Cover and boil for 10 minutes. Then simmer, uncovered, for 5 more minutes.

Filling. Cut dough into 4 equal pieces; flour the cutting board as necessary. Roll each piece into a circle, approximately 7 inches in diameter. Don't roll too thin or it will break. It should be ⅛-inch thick. Place circles of dough on cookie sheets covered with parchment paper.

Spoon an equal amount of the tomato sauce onto each circle. Place an equal amount of the onions and peppers on top of each. Dice chicken; separate into 4 equal portions and place each onto calzones. Fold the dough over and pinch the edges together to get the classic calzone shape. Paint egg whites over top of each and cut a small "x" on top surface to let steam escape.

Bake for 30 minutes.

Makes 4 Servings

NUTRITION PER SERVING Calories = 400								
	Total Fat	Sat. Fat	Poly. Fat	Mono. Fat	Carbs	Fiber	Sugars	Protein
grams	3.6 g	0.7 g	1.4 g	0.6	63.4 g	11.5 g	9.6 g	34 g
% of calories	8%				59%			33%

CHICKEN PICCATA, ASPARAGUS, AND RED POTATOES

Chicken Piccata is, by far, one of my favorite dishes for easy and satisfying entertaining. Spices are what make this dish so tasty: capers, lemon, rosemary, thyme, and parsley combine perfectly to create a wonderful flavor that will have your guests wanting seconds!

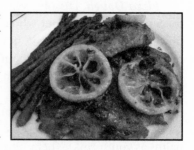

Ingredients

4 cups diced small red potatoes
Canola oil cooking spray
3 tablespoons rosemary
3 tablespoons thyme
$^1/_3$ cup whole-wheat flour
½ teaspoon salt
½ teaspoon pepper
2 whole eggs
1 pound chicken breasts (four 4-ounce breasts)
1 clove garlic, minced

1 cup chicken broth—low sodium
¼ cup capers
⅛ cup lemon juice
1 cup white wine
1 lemon, thinly sliced
3 cups asparagus—ends snapped and cut
2 tablespoons fresh chopped parsley

Directions:

Potatoes. Preheat oven to 350°F. Spread a single layer of red potatoes evenly in a baking dish. Spray with a very light coating of canola oil. Evenly sprinkle rosemary and thyme over top. Bake for 45 minutes, misting them with oil and shaking them every 15 minutes to ensure they cook evenly. Five minutes before serving, broil potatoes to get them extra crispy.

Chicken. Mix whole-wheat flour, salt, and pepper and spread evenly in a shallow dish. Beat eggs in a wide bowl. Dip each breast into the eggs and then coat with a thin layer of wheat flour on all sides. Pat off excess flour.

Spray bottom of pan with 2-second spray of canola oil cooking spray. Set on medium heat. Add breasts to pan and cook until outsides of breasts are light brown (approximately 2–3 minutes on each side). Transfer to a platter and keep warm.

Using same pan, spray another 1-second spray of canola oil and add garlic. Cook for 30 seconds. Add chicken broth, capers, lemon juice, and cooking wine, and bring to a boil. Add chicken and put thin slices of lemon over chicken. Cover and reduce heat to a simmer. Cook for 10 minutes.

Asparagus. Bring water to a boil in a large pot. Add asparagus and cook until bright green. Remove from pot and drain. Run cold water over asparagus.

Serve potatoes, asparagus, and chicken together, and sprinkle the 2 tablespoons of parsley on top for presentation.

Makes 4 Servings

NUTRITION PER SERVING Calories = 352								
	Total Fat	Sat. Fat	Poly. Fat	Mono. Fat	Carbs	Fiber	Sugars	Protein
grams	9 g	1.5 g	1.2 g	3.6 g	42.8 g	6.1 g	5 g	27 g
% of calories	21%				45%			30%

* *Note that the total percentage of calories doesn't add up to 100 percent because approximately 4 percent comes from alcohol in the wine.*

CHICKEN, BROCCOLI, AND BROWN RICE

This is a well-balanced dish that stores beautifully for up to a week. Multiply the ingredients for several dinners or lunches.

Ingredients
¼ cup long-grain brown rice
3 ounces skinless chicken breast
½ cup chicken broth
½ teaspoon ginger—ground
1 clove garlic—minced
Salt and pepper to taste
2 cups broccoli flowerets
½ tablespoon extra-virgin olive oil
Parsley—fresh chopped
1 tablespoon low-sodium soy sauce

Directions: Preheat oven to 350°F. Combine rice with ½ cup of water in a small pot with a tight-fitting lid. Bring to a boil. Stir and cover. Reduce heat to simmer and cook for 50 minutes.

Put chicken in a baking dish and pour chicken broth over breast. Sprinkle with ginger, minced garlic, salt, and pepper. Bake chicken in oven for 20 minutes or until completely cooked through.

Wash broccoli under cold water. Steam broccoli for 3 to 5 minutes or until it turns bright green. When done, run under cool water.

Combine cooked rice with chicken and broccoli. Mix in olive oil, fresh parsley, and soy sauce. Stir thoroughly and serve in a bowl.

Makes 1 Serving

	Total Fat	Sat. Fat	Poly. Fat	Mono. Fat	Carbs	Fiber	Sugars	Protein
grams	9.8 g	1.6 g	1.5 g	5.7 g	50.2 g	6.5 g	4 g	29 g
% of calories	22%				50%			28%

NUTRITION PER SERVING — Calories = 398

SNACKS

Any of these snacks can be enjoyed in the morning or afternoon. They are meant to be lighter than your main meals (ranging from 100 to 270 calories each), but still balanced to keep you feeling satisfied throughout the day.

GARBANZO NUTS

Delightfully crunchy, full of protein, and perfect for an energy boost.

Ingredients
Canola oil cooking spray
Parchment paper
1 can chickpeas (15 ounces)—
    rinsed and drained
½ teaspoon cayenne pepper
3 teaspoons garlic powder
½ teaspoon cumin powder

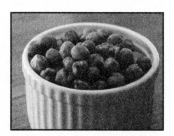

Directions: Preheat oven to 400°F. Spray light coating of canola oil onto cookie sheet covered in parchment paper. Mix chickpeas with spices and place in single layer on cookie sheet. Bake for approximately 40 minutes, stirring occasionally. When done, store in an airtight container to maintain crispness.

Makes 4 Servings

	Total Fat	Sat. Fat	Poly. Fat	Mono. Fat	Carbs	Fiber	Sugars	Protein
NUTRITION PER SERVING Calories = 138								
grams	2 g	0.3 g	0.7 g	1.1 g	24 g	4.7 g	0 g	5 g
% of calories	12%				74%			14%

SPICED TUNA ON CRACKERS

This is a great snack on whole-wheat crackers. Wasa crackers are only one option. Just make sure the crackers you use are made with whole grains and are high in fiber.

Ingredients

1 can solid white tuna—7 ounces (packed in spring water)
1 tablespoon Dijon mustard
2 teaspoons extra-virgin olive oil
1 teaspoon lemon juice

¼ teaspoon garlic powder
¼ teaspoon dried oregano
¼ teaspoon black pepper
Dash paprika
4 Wasa multigrain crackers
2 large romaine lettuce leaves

Directions: Drain tuna. In a bowl, mix tuna, mustard, olive oil, lemon juice, garlic, oregano, pepper, and paprika. Scoop an equal portion of tuna mixture onto 2 Wasa crackers and top each with a piece of romaine lettuce. Top each with another Wasa cracker to make 2 sandwiches.

Makes 2 Servings

NUTRITION PER SERVING Calories = 239								
	Total Fat	Sat. Fat	Poly. Fat	Mono. Fat	Carbs	Fiber	Sugars	Protein
grams	5.4 g	0.9 g	0.9 g	3.5 g	22.7 g	5.1 g	1 g	25.8 g
% of calories	20%				35%			45%

ARTICHOKE AND TANGY SAUCE

Naturally, you will eat artichokes slowly, leaf by leaf. They are full of fiber and vitamins, especially vitamin K. If you don't eat dairy, replace the yogurt with one package of silken tofu. The nutritional information will vary minimally.

Ingredients
4 fresh artichokes (1 per serving)

Ingredients—Sauce

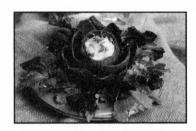

2 green onions—
   finely chopped
1½ cups plain nonfat
   Greek yogurt
2 tablespoons lemon juice
2 tablespoons Dijon mustard
1 tablespoon fresh tarragon
¼ cup fresh parsley—finely chopped
1 clove garlic—minced
½ teaspoon salt
½ teaspoon black pepper

Directions: Place washed artichokes in a closed casserole dish with approximately 2 cups of water. Microwave on high for about 15 minutes. Wiggle the leaves, and if they are not loose, microwave for another 10 minutes, or until they are soft and flexible.

    Sauce. While artichoke is cooking, blend all other ingredients in a food processor. Dip the artichoke leaves in the sauce and enjoy!

Makes 4 Servings—2 cups of sauce

NUTRITION PER SERVING								
Calories = 114								
	Total Fat	Sat. Fat	Poly. Fat	Mono. Fat	Carbs	Fiber	Sugars	Protein
grams	0.8 g	0.1 g	0.3 g	0.2 g	18.9 g	10.9 g	4 g	11 g
% of calories	6%				60%			34%

EDAMAME

Edamame is a well-balanced, easy-to-prepare, tasty snack. Not only is it fun to eat, but because the beans are in pods, you eat them slowly, giving your stomach time to realize that it is getting full. When possible, choose organic, non-GMO (genetically modified organisms) edamame!

Ingredients
2 cups unshelled edamame pods (or 1 cup shelled)

Directions: Microwave for 30 seconds on medium for a light steaming. Eat the beans!

Makes 1 Serving

	Total Fat	Sat. Fat	Poly. Fat	Mono. Fat	Carbs	Fiber	Sugars	Protein
NUTRITION PER SERVING Calories = 189								
grams	8.1 g	1 g	3.3 g	2.0 g	15.8 g	8.1 g	3.4 g	17 g
% of calories	36%				33%			31%

BANANA AND ALMOND BUTTER

Ingredients

1 banana
1 tablespoon all-natural almond butter

Directions: Cut banana into ½-inch slices and dip into almond butter.

Makes 1 Serving

	Total Fat	Sat. Fat	Poly. Fat	Mono. Fat	Carbs	Fiber	Sugars	Protein
NUTRITION PER SERVING Calories = 206								
grams	9.8 g	1.0 g	2.1 g	6.2 g	30.3 g	4 g	14.4 g	4 g
% of calories	40%				54%			6%

GREEN BEAN, FETA, AND WALNUT SALAD

This salad has great crunch and flavor. The walnuts provide a good dose of heart-healthy fats, while the fat-free feta gives you protein!

Ingredients

1 medium yellow onion—
finely chopped
1 tablespoon extra-virgin
olive oil
4 cups green beans

¼ cup fat-free feta
1/8 cup finely chopped walnuts
1 teaspoon salt
1 teaspoon pepper

Directions: Lightly sauté onions with a teaspoon of olive oil until translucent. Steam green beans until dark green—just al dente. When done, mix green beans, feta, chopped walnuts, and sautéed onions in a medium-size bowl. Add remaining olive oil (2 teaspoons), salt, and pepper, and toss until well mixed. Store unused portion in a tightly sealed container to preserve freshness and crunch!

Makes 2 Servings

NUTRITION PER SERVING Calories = 241							
	Total Fat	Sat. Fat	Poly. Fat	Mono. Fat	Carbs	Fiber	Sugars	Protein
grams	11.8 g	1.5 g	4.3 g	5.6 g	23 g	9 g	6 g	14 g
% of calories	42%				37%			21%

MEDITERRANEAN CHICKPEA SALAD

Chickpeas are loaded with fiber and are a good source of protein. You can make this salad with any type of bean, although chickpeas are especially tasty. This salad makes a great side dish or midday snack.

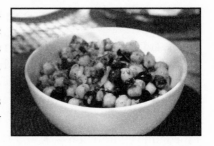

Ingredients
1 can chickpeas (15 ounces)—drained and rinsed
½ yellow onion—finely chopped
¼ cup chopped black olives
¼ cup jarred roasted sweet red peppers—chopped
1 teaspoon fresh basil—minced
2 tablespoons chopped garlic
½ tablespoon extra-virgin olive oil
2 tablespoons balsamic vinegar
Salt and pepper to taste

Directions: Combine chickpeas, onion, olives, roasted peppers, basil, and garlic, and mix well. Add olive oil, balsamic vinegar, salt, and pepper. Mix thoroughly and serve at room temperature or chilled.

Makes 4 Servings

NUTRITION PER SERVING Calories = 175								
	Total Fat	Sat. Fat	Poly. Fat	Mono. Fat	Carbs	Fiber	Sugars	Protein
grams	3.9 g	0.5 g	0.8 g	2.2 g	29.6 g	5.6 g	2 g	6 g
% of calories	19%				69%			12%

PERFECT-FOR-SNACKING COUSCOUS

Ingredients
2 cups dried black lentils
1 cup whole-grain couscous—uncooked
¾ teaspoon salt (¼ teaspoon and ½ teaspoon)
1 cup cherry tomatoes—quartered
1 cup dried apricot—coarsely chopped
²/₃ cup red onion—finely chopped
¹/₃ cup cucumber, unpeeled—finely chopped
¼ cup fresh parsley—chopped
3 tablespoons fresh mint—chopped
3 tablespoons fresh lemon juice
1 tablespoon extra-virgin olive oil
½ cup feta cheese—crumbled

Directions: Rinse lentils in cold water and drain. Place 4 cups of water into a large saucepan, add lentils, and bring to a boil. Reduce heat and simmer for 20 minutes or until soft. Drain.

Bring 1 cup of water to a boil in a medium saucepan. Add couscous and ¼ teaspoon salt. Remove from heat, cover, and let stand for 5 minutes. Fluff with a fork. Combine couscous with tomatoes, apricot, onion, cucumber, parsley, mint, lemon juice, remaining salt, and oil, and gently mix. Top with feta and serve.

Makes 8 Servings

NUTRITION PER SERVING Calories = 234							
	Total Fat	Sat. Fat	Poly. Fat	Mono. Fat	Carbs	Fiber	Sugars	Protein
grams	4.2 g	1.7 g	0.4 g	1.7 g	41 g	7 g	12 g	10 g
% of calories	16%				69%			15%

GAZPACHO, SHRIMP, AND TOAST

Gazpacho is a delicious cold soup. Coupled with a few shrimp and a slice of whole-grain bread, it provides a healthy dose of fiber and protein to keep you feeling satisfied.

Ingredients

1 medium onion
1 long cucumber
2 medium tomatoes
½ red pepper
½ green pepper
Tomato sauce (16 ounces)
8 ounces chicken or vegetable
  broth

¼ cup red wine vinegar
Salt and pepper to taste
1 clove garlic—minced
Tabasco sauce to taste
12 medium-sized shrimp
  (3 per serving)
4 slices whole-grain bread
  (1 per serving)

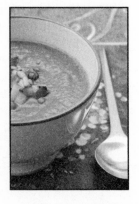

Directions: Cut vegetables into medium-size pieces and blend them in a food processor until very fine. Pour mixture into bowl and add tomato sauce, chicken broth, vinegar, salt, pepper, garlic, and Tabasco sauce. Blend and chill.

To serve: Clean, devein, and boil shrimp until cooked; toast bread. Serve soup chilled with 3 shrimp and 1 piece of toast per serving.

Makes 4 Servings

	Total Fat	Sat. Fat	Poly. Fat	Mono. Fat	Carbs	Fiber	Sugars	Protein
NUTRITION PER SERVING Calories = 164								
grams	2 g	0.4 g	0.8 g	0.3 g	27.8 g	6 g	11 g	11 g
% of calories	11%				65%			24%

BRAN MUFFINS

Sucanat is made from sugar cane; however, it retains more nutritional value than brown sugar. With the use of whole-wheat flour and wheat bran to boost the fiber content, these muffins are a sweet AND filling snack or breakfast!

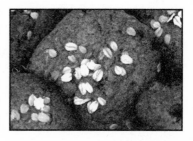

Ingredients

¾ cup unbleached all-purpose flour
½ cup whole-wheat flour
1¼ cups natural wheat bran
¾ cup Sucanat (brown sugar can be used instead)
1 tablespoon baking powder
1 teaspoon baking soda
¼ teaspoon cinnamon
¼ teaspoon nutmeg
¼ teaspoon salt
1 egg
1¼ cups plain nonfat Greek yogurt
2 tablespoons canola oil
3½ teaspoons vanilla extract
1 cup whole golden raisins
Muffin/cupcake liners

Directions: Preheat oven to 375°F. In large bowl, blend flours, bran, Sucanat, baking powder, baking soda, cinnamon, nutmeg, and salt. In smaller bowl, beat egg and mix in yogurt, oil, and vanilla. Make an indentation in center of dry ingredients and pour in egg mixture. Fold in raisins, just until dry ingredients are moistened. Pour mixture into prelined muffin trays. Bake for 20 to 25 minutes.

Makes 12 Servings

NUTRITION PER SERVING Calories = 193								
	Total Fat	Sat. Fat	Poly. Fat	Mono. Fat	Carbs	Fiber	Sugars	Protein
Grams	3 g	0.5 g	0.5 g	1.9 g	38.8 g	4 g	23 g	5 g
% of calories	15%				75%			10%

HEARTS AND MOONS CHERRY AND CELERY SALAD

Ingredients

1 cup sliced celery
1 cup cherries—pitted and halved
1 cup sugar snap peas, shelled
3 tablespoons chopped fresh parsley

¼ cup plain nonfat Greek yogurt
1 tablespoon pecans—chopped
1½ teaspoons fresh lemon juice
Salt and pepper to taste

Directions: Combine all ingredients. Serve well chilled.

Makes 3 Servings

NUTRITION PER SERVING Calories = 132								
	Total Fat	Sat. Fat	Poly. Fat	Mono. Fat	Carbs	Fiber	Sugars	Protein
grams	7 g	0.6 g	2.0 g	4.2 g	14 g	3 g	10 g	5 g
% of calories	46%				39%			15%

APPLE, WALNUTS, AND YOGURT

Ingredients

$^1/_8$ cup chopped walnuts
½ cup plain nonfat Greek
   yogurt

1 teaspoon honey
1 apple—cored and chopped

Directions: Lightly mix ingredients together and enjoy.

Makes 1 Serving

NUTRITION PER SERVING Calories = 272								
	Total Fat	Sat. Fat	Poly. Fat	Mono. Fat	Carbs	Fiber	Sugars	Protein
grams	9.5 g	0.6 g	5.5 g	2.3 g	36.9 g	5.4 g	29 g	16 g
% of calories	29%				49%			22%

CARROTS AND HUMMUS

Hummus is very easy to make and can be stored up to one week. Tahini can be found in Middle Eastern groceries or in the international food section of grocery stores. If you can't find tahini, you can substitute one tablespoon of sesame oil for the paste. Carrots, snow peas, and endive are great dipping vegetables, but you can use any you like.

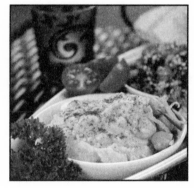

Ingredients

1 can chickpeas (15 ounces)— drained and rinsed

4 tablespoons lemon juice

2 tablespoons extra-virgin olive oil

2 tablespoons sesame tahini (sesame paste)

1 tablespoon paprika

4 cloves garlic

6 cups baby carrots (you can use broccoli, cauliflower, peppers, and celery; for 1 serving, use only 1 cup)

Directions: Blend chickpeas, lemon juice, olive oil, tahini, paprika, and garlic in a food processor until smooth and creamy.

Makes 6 Servings

NUTRITION PER SERVING Calories = 215								
	Total Fat	Sat. Fat	Poly. Fat	Mono. Fat	Carbs	Fiber	Sugars	Protein
grams	8.2 g	1.1 g	2.1 g	4.4 g	32 g	7.7 g	6 g	6 g
% of calories	33%				58%			9%

CHIC CUCUMBER SANDWICH

This is a far cry from your grandmother's finger sandwiches!

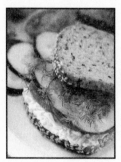

Ingredients

2 slices 100% whole-grain bread

½ cup nonfat plain Greek yogurt

Dash of dill

Dash of pepper

Sprinkle of lemon juice

¼ cup cucumber—thinly sliced

¼ cup tomato—thinly sliced

Directions: Toast bread. Spread yogurt onto 1 slice and sprinkle with dill, pepper, and lemon juice. Top with cucumber slices, tomato, and second slice of bread.

Makes 1 Serving

	Total Fat	Sat. Fat	Poly. Fat	Mono. Fat	Carbs	Fiber	Sugars	Protein
	NUTRITION PER SERVING Calories = 218							
grams	2 g	0.4 g	0.4 g	0.9 g	31.1 g	4.5 g	9.5 g	20 g
% of calories	8%				56%			36%

DESSERTS

Desserts are a treat, worth the indulgence once in a while. The following recipes provide options that are healthier than most, without sacrificing taste. Although some of the ingredients are atypical to the "GET REAL" principles (such as the use of a small amount of butter), most ingredients are healthy and nutritious.

DATE TRUFFLES

Truffles are a great mini-dessert when entertaining. Be careful, though; they easily pop in your mouth, so don't become too addicted!

Ingredients
¼ cup almonds—finely chopped
20 dates—pitted
1 tablespoon honey
1 teaspoon vanilla extract
2 tablespoons cocoa powder—dry and unsweetened

Directions: Preheat oven to 400°F. Roast almonds for 6 minutes or until lightly toasted. Dice dates and mix in honey, vanilla, and almonds in a food processor. Shape batter into quarter-sized balls and roll in cocoa powder. Freeze for at least 15 minutes to solidify before eating.

Makes 12 Truffles (Serving Size = 2 Truffles)

NUTRITION PER SERVING Calories = 272								
	Total Fat	Sat. Fat	Poly. Fat	Mono. Fat	Carbs	Fiber	Sugars	Protein
grams	3.4 g	0.4 g	0.7 g	2.0 g	65.1 g	6.6 g	56.4 g	3 g
% of calories	10%				86%			4%

ANGEL FOOD LAYER CAKE FROM HEAVEN

A slice of this cake will remind you of heaven! I love making this dessert for guests because it is easy, delicious, and beautiful. It's also low in fat and offers a bit of protein. It is a great way to end a fun-filled evening with friends—just get ready for lots of compliments.

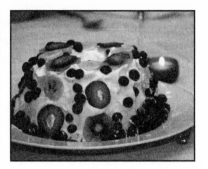

Ingredients

¾ cup whole-wheat flour or whole-wheat pastry flour
1¼ cups sugar
¼ cup cornstarch
12 large egg whites—room temperature
½ teaspoon salt
1½ teaspoons cream of tartar
2 teaspoons almond extract
Angel food cake pan
2½ cups Truwhip topping*
1 kiwi—peeled and cut crosswise into ⅛-inch slices
½ cup strawberries—stemmed and cut lengthwise into ⅛-inch slices
½ cup blueberries
1 small banana—cut into ⅛-inch slices

Directions:

Cake. Preheat oven to 325°F. Blend whole-wheat flour in food processor until very fine (if using whole-wheat pastry flour, you don't need to do this). Sift together finely blended flour, ¾ cup of the sugar, and cornstarch in a bowl. Set aside.

Beat egg whites, salt, and cream of tartar until they form soft peaks. Gradually, add remaining ½ cup of sugar and almond extract, and beat until mixed. Gently fold in flour mixture, one-third at a time. Pour into angel food cake pan and bake for 1 hour or until cake is springy when poked. Remove from oven and invert cake to cool. Allow it to cool completely before removing from pan.

Decoration. Defrost Truwhip in refrigerator for 4 hours prior to decorating (do not microwave). Once cake is completely cooled from baking, remove from pan and cut in half to create an upper layer and a lower layer.

Using a spatula, evenly apply a layer of truwhip onto the top of cake's lower layer.

Take a portion of the kiwi, strawberries, blueberries, and bananas, and place into truwhip to create a single layer of fruit. Place upper layer of cake on top. Use rest of truwhip to evenly coat sides and top of cake. When done, use remainder of kiwi, strawberries, blueberries, and banana to decorate cake on the top and sides, creating a beautiful, colorful, and tasty dessert.

Store any unused portion in a sealed container and refrigerate.

Makes 12 Servings

	Total Fat	Sat. Fat	Poly. Fat	Mono. Fat	Carbs	Fiber	Sugars	Protein
NUTRITION PER SERVING Calories = 200								
grams	3.6 g	3.4 g	0.1 g	0 g	38 g	2 g	27 g	5 g
% of calories	18%				72%			9%

* Truwhip is an all-natural whipped topping that has zero trans fats, no hydrogenated oils, and no GMOs, making it a better product than other whipped toppings.

GRANDMA'S CHOCOLATE CLUSTERS

Dark chocolate has been proven to deliver antioxidants and other healthful benefits. The good news is that it also tastes fabulous. These clusters are low in fat, have some protein, and are a good source of fiber. If you are absolutely against tofu, you can substitute an equal amount of low-fat cream cheese.

Ingredients
½ cup chopped walnuts
100 grams dark chocolate (at least 70% cacao)
150 grams silken tofu—soft
1 cup raisins
16 ounces whole-wheat pretzels—crushed

Directions: Preheat the oven to 300°F. Toast walnuts for 7 minutes. Melt chocolate in double boiler, stirring so it is melted through. Whip tofu by hand until smooth, pour in chocolate and mix well. Add in walnuts, raisins, and pretzels, and mix so they are all well coated in the chocolate mixture. Place tablespoon-sized spoonfuls onto a cookie sheet lined with wax paper. Freeze clusters for at least an hour before serving.

Makes 12 Servings

	Total Fat	Sat. Fat	Poly. Fat	Mono. Fat	Carbs	Fiber	Sugars	Protein
NUTRITION PER SERVING Calories = 265								
grams	8.1 g	2.6 g	2.9 g	2.0 g	46 g	4.6 g	10 g	7 g
% of calories	27%				64%			9%

SUMMER'S OVER APPLE CRUMBLE

You can use any in-season fruit to make this recipe work year-round. For a creamy texture, add a dollop of nonfat Greek yogurt on top.

Ingredients—Filling

3 cups Granny Smith apples— sliced

2 cups raspberries (fresh if possible)

¾ cup whole-wheat flour

½ teaspoon cream of tartar

1 tablespoon cinnamon

1 tablespoon fennel seeds— crushed

Ingredients—Crumble

2½ cups old-fashioned rolled oats

1 teaspoon salt

2 tablespoons honey

4 tablespoons butter

Canola oil cooking spray

Directions: Preheat oven to 400°F. Combine apples and raspberries in large bowl. Add flour, cream of tartar, cinnamon, and fennel, and mix so the fruit is well covered. In separate bowl, combine oats and salt. Mix in honey and butter so it remains chunky and uneven. (DON'T over mix!)

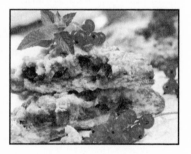

Spray a 9×9-inch ovenproof dish with canola oil cooking spray and pour in fruit filling. Cover with oat crumble on top. Bake for 20–25 minutes or until topping is nicely browned.

Makes 10 Servings

NUTRITION PER SERVING Calories = 272								
	Total Fat	Sat. Fat	Poly. Fat	Mono. Fat	Carbs	Fiber	Sugars	Protein
grams	7.7 g	3.4 g	1.4 g	2.1 g	45 g	8.4 g	8.5 g	8 g
% of calories	24%				65%			11%

FRUIT AND HONEY-MINT YOGURT SAUCE

This dessert is light, flavorful, and refreshing. The mint and lemon give it a nice little bite!

Ingredients
1 cup plain nonfat Greek yogurt
1 teaspoon lemon juice
1 tablespoon lemon zest
3 tablespoons honey
1 cup blueberries
1 cup strawberries—stemmed and sliced
1 large kiwi—peeled and sliced
1 cup red seedless grapes—cut in half
2 cups honeydew—cut into 1-inch cubes
3 tablespoons fresh mint—coarsely chopped
4 mint sprigs

Directions: In a small bowl, combine the yogurt, lemon juice, lemon zest, and honey. Stir until smooth.

In a large bowl, combine the blueberries, strawberries, kiwi, grapes, and honeydew. Sprinkle the mint over the fruit and toss gently. Pour the yogurt mixture over the top and toss until the fruit is evenly coated. Use mint sprigs for garnish.

Makes 4 Servings

	Total Fat	Sat. Fat	Poly. Fat	Mono. Fat	Carbs	Fiber	Sugars	Protein
NUTRITION PER SERVING Calories = 189								
grams	0.6 g	0.1 g	0.3 g	0.2 g	42.5 g	4 g	36 g	8 g
% of calories	3%				81%			16%

ABOUT THE AUTHOR

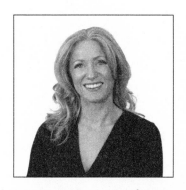

Brett Blumenthal earned her bachelor's degree and an MBA from Cornell University. She is a WELCOA-certified wellness expert and AFAA-certified fitness instructor who previously taught at Cornell, Gold's Gym, and Bally Total Fitness. Two decades of experience in the wellness industry and over ten years of experience in management consulting inspired her to found Sheer Balance in 2007, and most recently, the Healthy Road Warrior in 2010, both with the goal of helping people find balance and health easily, naturally, and sustainably. She is a regular guest speaker at conferences, expos, and wellness centers around the world and consults with individuals, corporations, and wellness organizations on business strategy, health, and wellness. Her writing is regularly featured on such popular Web sites as Yahoo!, Shine from Yahoo!, Divine Caroline, Intent, Wellsphere, Tonic, and Gather. She has received numerous awards for Sheer Balance and her influential blogging.

REFERENCES

CHAPTER 1

Bray, G. A., S. J. Nielsen, and B. M. Popkin. 2004. Consumption of high-fructose corn syrup in beverages may play a role in the epidemic of obesity. *American Journal of Clinical Nutrition* 79: 537–43.

Bruce, B., G. A. Spiller, L. M. Klevay, and S. K. Gallagher. 2000. A diet high in whole and unrefined foods favorably alters lipids, antioxidant defenses, and colon function. *Journal of the American College of Nutrition* 19: 61–67.

Centers for Disease Control and Prevention (CDC). How to use fruits and vegetables to help manage your weight. http://www.cdc.gov/healthyweight/healthy_eating/fruits vegetables.html. Accessed August 2, 2009.

Cornell University Food and Brand Lab. Can "low-fat" nutrition labels lead to obesity? http://foodpsychology.cornell.edu/research/overeat/index.htm. Accessed August 3, 2009.

Feingold Association of the United States. Artificial flavors. http://www.feingold.org/pg-overview.html. Accessed August 7, 2009.

Fowler, S. P., K. Williams, R. G. Resendez, K. J. Hunt, H. P. Hazuda, and M. P. Stern. 2008. Fueling the obesity epidemic? Artificially sweetened beverage use and long-term weight gain. *Obesity* (Silver Spring) 16: 1894–1900.

Harvard School of Public Health. The nutrition source. http://www.hsph.harvard.edu. Accessed August 1, 2009.

Harvard School of Public Health. Separating the whole grain from the chaff. https://apps.sph.harvard.edu. Accessed August 8, 2009.

Healing with Whole Foods. Upcoming event description. http://www.healingwithwholefoods.com. Accessed August 2, 2009.

Internet FAQ Archive. Nutrient health claims. http://www.faqs.org/nutrition/Foo-Hea/Health-Claims.html. Accessed August 1, 2009.

Jiménez-Monreal, A. M., L. García-Diz M. Martínez-Tomé, M. Mariscal, and M. A. Murcia. 2009. Influence of cooking methods on antioxidant activity of vegetables. *Journal of Food Science* 74(3): H97–H103.

Mayo Clinic. Healthy cooking techniques: Sautéing. http://mayoclinic.com/health/healthy-cooking/NU00201. Accessed August 6, 2009.

Metcalfe, D. D., and R. A. Simon. 2003. *Food Allergy: Adverse Reactions to Foods and Food Additives.* Blackwell 3: 388.

Miglio, C., E. Chiavaro, A. Visconti, V. Fogliano, and N. Pellegrini. 2008. Effects of different cooking methods on nutritional and physiochemical characteristics of selected vegetables. *Journal of Agricultural and Food Chemistry* 56(1): 139–47.

Parker-Pope, T. 2008. Finding the best way to cook all those vegetables. *New York Times.*

Swithers, S. E., and T. L. Davidson. 2008. A role for sweet taste: calorie predictive relations in energy regulation by rats. *Behavioral Neuroscience* 122: 161–73.

United States Department of Agriculture (USDA). MyPyramid: What foods are in the grain groups? http://www.mypyramid. gov/pyramid/grains.html. Accessed August 1, 2009.

United States Food and Drug Administration (FDA). Definitions of nutrient content claims. http://www.fda.gov/Food/GuidanceComplianceRegulatoryInformation/GuidanceDocuments/FoodLabelingNutrition/FoodLabelingGuide/default. htm. Accessed August 1, 2009.

United States Food and Drug Administration (FDA). Listing of food additive status. http://www.fda.gov/Food/FoodIngredientsPackaging/FoodAdditives/FoodAdditiveListings/ ucm091048.htm. Accessed August 8, 2009.

Weston A. Price Foundation. Wise traditions in food, farming, and the healing arts. http://www.westonaprice.org. Accessed August 1, 2009.

Wilkins, J.L., J.C. Bokaer-Smith, and D. Hilchey. 1996. Local foods and local agriculture: A survey of attitudes among Northeastern consumers. *A Survey of Northeast Consumers.*

Willett, W. C. 2001. *Eat, Drink, and Be Healthy.* New York: Free Press.

CHAPTER 2

Fruits & Veggies More Matters. Healthy cooking with fruits and vegetables. http://www.fruitsandveggiesmorematters. org/?page_id=5. Accessed August 3, 2009.

Harvard School of Public Health. The nutrition source: What should you eat? http://www.hsph.harvard.edu/nutrition-source/what-should-you-eat/pyramid/. Accessed August 1, 2009.

Howarth, N. C., E. Saltzman, and S. B. Roberts. 2001. Dietary fiber and weight regulation. *Nutrition Review* 59: 129–39.

Mayo Clinic. Healthy cooking techniques: Sautéing. http://mayoclinic.com/health/healthy-cooking/NU0020. Accessed August 6, 2009.

Roberts, S. B., M. A. McCrory, and E. Saltzman. 2002. The influence of dietary composition on energy intake and body weight. *Journal of the American College of Nutrition* 21(2): 140S–145S.

Schroeder, N., D. D. Gallaher, E. A. Arndt, and L. Marquart. 2009. Influence of whole grain barley, whole grain wheat, and refined rice-based foods on short-term satiety and energy intake. *Appetite* 53(3): 363–369.

Willett, W. C. 2001. *Eat, Drink, and Be Healthy*. New York: Free Press.

United States Department of Agriculture (USDA). MyPyramid: Inside the pyramid. http://www.mypyramid.gov. Accessed August 8, 2009.

CHAPTER 3

Harvard School of Public Health. The nutrition source: What should you eat? http://www.hsph.harvard.edu/nutrition-source/what-should-you-eat/pyramid/. Accessed August 8, 2009.

Halton, T. L., W. C. Willett, S. Liu, et al. 2006. Low-carbohydrate-diet score and the risk of coronary heart disease in women. *New England Journal of Medicine* 355: 1991–2002.

Hoffman, J. R., and M. J. Falvo. 2004. Protein—which is best? *Journal of Sports Science and Medicine* 3: 118–30.

Jancurova, M., L. Minarovicova, and A. Dander. 2009. Quinoa: A review. *Czech Journal of Food Sciences* 27(2): 71–79.

Layman, D. K., E. L. Evans, D. Erickson, J. Seyler, J. Weber, D. Bagshaw, A. Griel, T. Psota, and P. Kris-Etherton. 2009. A moderate-protein diet produces sustained weight loss and long-term changes in body composition and blood lipids in obese adults. *The Journal of Nutrition* 139(3): 514–521.

Mayo Clinic. Healthy cooking techniques: Sautéing. http://mayoclinic.com/health/healthy-cooking/NU00201. Accessed August 6, 2009.

Sacks, F. M., A. Lichtenstein, L. Van Horn, W. Harris, P. Kris-Etherton, and M. Winston. 2006. Soy protein, isoflavones, and cardiovascular health: An American Heart Association science advisory for professionals from the nutrition committee. *Circulation* 113: 1034–1044.

Somer, E., and N. Snyderman. 1999. *Food & Mood: The Complete Guide to Eating Well and Feeling Your Best.* New York: Holt Paperbacks.

United States Department of Agriculture (USDA). MyPyramid: Inside the pyramid. http://www.mypyramid.gov/pyramid/index.html. Accessed August 8, 2009.

Willett, W. C. 2001. *Eat, Drink, and Be Healthy.* New York: Free Press.

CHAPTER 4

Harvard School of Public Health. The nutrition source: What should you eat? http://www.hsph.harvard.edu/nutrition-source/what-should-you-eat/pyramid/. Accessed August 8, 2009.

Hu, F. B., J. E. Manson, and W. C. Willett. 2001. Types of dietary fat and risk of coronary heart disease: a critical review. *Journal of the American College of Nutrition* 20: 5–19.

Michaels, J., C. Darwin, and M. V. Aalst. 2009. *Master Your Metabolism: The 3 Diet Secrets to Naturally Balancing Your Hormones for a Hot and Healthy Body!* New York: Random House, Inc.

Willett, W. C. 2001. *Eat, Drink, and Be Healthy*. New York: Free Press.

CHAPTER 5

Raynor, H. A., H. M. Niemeier, and R. R. Wing. 2006. Effect of limiting snack food variety on long-term sensory-specific satiety and monotony during obesity treatment. *Eating Behaviors* 7: 1–14.

Small Plate Movement. About SPM. http://www.smallplatemovement.org. Accessed August 1, 2009.

Wansink, B. 2006. *Mindless Eating: Why We Eat More Than We Think*. New York: Bantam Dell.

OTHER RESOURCES

- American Heart Association: www.americanheart.org
- Ban Trans Fats: The Campaign to Ban Partially Hydrogenated Oils: www.bantransfats.com
- The Center for Mindful Eating: www.tcme.org
- Center for Science in the Public Interest: www.cspinet.org
- Consumer Health Reviews: www.consumerhealthreviews.com
- Feingold Association of the United States: www.feingold.org
- Harvard School of Public Health: www.hsph.harvard.edu
- Institute of Food Science and Technology: www.ifst.org
- My Pyramid: www.mypyramid.gov
- National Cancer Institute: www.cancer.gov
- National Center for Biotechnology Information: www.ncbi.nih.gov
- Natural News: www.newstarget.com
- Nutrition Data: www.nutritiondata.com
- Whole Grains Council: www.wholegrainscouncil.org